MIND-BODY
HARMONY

HOW TO RESIST AND RECOVER FROM AUTOIMMUNE DISEASES

Terry Willard CIH, Ph.D.

Mary T. Kelly, MA

Foreword by Hyla Cass, MD

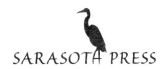

SARASOTA PRESS

National Library of Canada Cataloguing-in-Publication Data

Willard, Terry, 1951–

Resisting and recovering from auto-immune diseases / Terry Willard.

Includes index.

ISBN 1-55356-016-7

1. Autoimmune diseases—Popular works. I. Title.

RS164.W534 2003   616.97'8   C2003-900328-0

THE CANADA COUNCIL   LE CONSEIL DES ARTS
FOR THE ARTS   DU CANADA
SINCE 1957   DEPUIS 1957

ONTARIO ARTS COUNCIL
CONSEIL DES ARTS DE L'ONTARIO

The publisher gratefully acknowledges the support of the Canada Council for the Arts and
the Ontario Arts Council for its publishing program.

We acknowledge the financial support of the Government of Canada through the Book
Publishing Industry Development Program (BPIDP) for our publishing activities.

We acknowledge the support of the Government of Ontario through the Ontario Media
Development Corporation's Ontario Book Initiative.

Sarasota Press is an imprint of
Key Porter Books Limited
70 The Esplanade
Toronto, Ontario
Canada M5E 1R4

www.keyporter.com

*Publisher's Note: The contents of the book are not intended to be used as a substitution for consultation
with your physician or health care practitioner. All matters pertaining to your health should be directed
to a health care professional.*

Design: Jack Steiner
Electronic formatting: Heidy Lawrance Associates

Printed and bound in Canada

03 04 05 06 07 08 6 5 4 3 2 1

Dedication

✤

This book is dedicated to all of our higher-selves. May we collectively connect with our causal bodies to heal ourselves and to bring everlasting peace to our mother, Gaia. Special thanks go to the devas that have, and are, helping in this process. A particular dedication goes to Vanya, Damon, Aiyana, Yarrow and Juniper, for the closeness and love you have shown me and this process.

Acknowledgements

✤

The numbers of people that have contributed to the process of this book are too numerous to list as they extend over twenty years and many discussions. I thank you all, as you know who you are. A particular thanks goes to Dr. Hyla Cass, whose long initial discussions contributed to the birth of this book. The diagrams that my lovely daughter, Aiyana helped create deserve special mention. I would like to thank all the readers that have labored over the many rewrites of this book; your contributions have been great. Again I thank the fine people at Key Porter books, with special thanks to Janice Zawerbny, Paula Chabanais, and Clare McKeon.

CONTENTS

Foreword

Terry Willard takes us on a fascinating journey of discovery regarding the nature health and disease. Based on the concepts of "energetic" or "vibrational" medicine, his application of this relatively new area to the use of botanical remedies and their energetics is novel and intriguing. In my own practice of holistic psychiatry, I have seen and puzzled over many of the same issues as Terry has. I was excited to find his elegant road map through mind, body, and spirit, revealing the energetic basis of imbalance, and providing original solutions using familiar remedies that can be found in your local health food store.

Terry begins by describing the various "bodies" —physical, emotional (astral), and mental, with the physical body comprising only one-seventh of who we really are! So, opposed to the commonly held beliefs about physical reality, "we are, in fact, spiritual beings having a physical experience." In turn, we see that plants too are more than just physical entities. By our "tuning" into their more etheric vibrations, we can choose the correct plant that can then resonate with our emotional and physical blocks, with profound healing effects.

This book uses the ever-expanding field of psychoneurimmunology (PNI), which is the relationship between the mind, the nervous system and the immune systems. It then explains how various forms of stress affect the PNI and can lead to autoimmune disease. However, the theories found here can apply to a much larger range of health issues, as well.

From a practitioner's point of view, we have to understand where the center of gravity of the health issue lies. Is it physical, emotional, or in one of the other subtle bodies? To elicit clues on how to treat a person, we use the acupuncture meridians and chakras, which function as communication lenses that focus their energies in the various bodies. Many people have emotional blocks or stored traumas that show up as "emotional miasms" that block the flow in these various subtle energy systems, leading to disease. By dislodging them, using a variety of techniques, from herbal medicine and homeopathy to energy psychology techniques (such as EMDR and Thought Field Therapy) we can speed up the healing process.

As Terry so clearly describes in both his detailed plant descriptions and in case histories, we can use botanicals simply as raw material for a chemical needed in the physical body. On the other hand, herbs can often be just as effective on an energetic level, to entrain the various bodies to move into a more balanced state. I am inspired by this more comprehensive approach to the use of herbal products, one that explains the miraculous dance that occurs in the invisible realms, both within us and between ourselves and the natural world. I am especially fascinated by his description of medicinal mushrooms, and see them and other plants as our natural healers on many levels. As Terry says, "Reishi is the best herb I have ever found to reduce brain chatter, repetitive thinking or circular arguments. For those cerebral types who live too much in their head, this herb is excellent." I hope we will see a more extensive list of botanicals addressed in this way in the near future.

For those without a solid basis in the fields of vibrational medicine, PNI, stress, and autoimmune disease, the first part of the book provides a solid background theory. Others may want to skip to part three, where specific treatment protocols provide the clinically practical part of the book.

Sit back and be prepared for some novel and even controversial ways of looking at the process of disease and healing, and certainly, a more comprehensive view of the effects of many herbal remedies. Well-illustrated by detailed and fascinating case histories, this book will intrigue, inspire, and maybe even change you in some mysterious way.

Hyla Cass, MD
Assistant Clinical Professor of Psychiatry,
UCLA School of Medicine
Author of *Natural Highs: Supplements, Nutrition,*
and *Mind/Body Techniques to Feel Good All the Time*

Introduction

✣

I started in clinical practice as a herbalist in the early 1970s; at that time most of the patients were either from the "counter culture" or from ethnic groups that used botanical remedies in their culture. By the late 1980s, herbal medicine had spilled into mainstream society. Now, the clients who walk through the door of our busy urban clinic are no different from those who visit any general practitioner, whether that be a naturopath, medical doctor or acupuncturist. Our clinic has fifteen natural health practitioners, all with different specialties and types of training; suffice it to say we see many people on a weekly basis. During the last two decades, not only has the type and number of our patients changed, so too has the nature of the health issues they present.

Having a large clinic with diverse practitioners gives us the advantage of being able to spot health trends as they emerge. During the last ten years or so, one of the major developments that we have seen is a dramatic increase in autoimmune issues, including chronic fatigue syndrome, fibromyalgia, irritable bowel syndrome and allergies to mention a few. This increase prompted me to ask two major questions. Why the increase in these types of disorders, and what are suitable protocols to treat these health issues?

Those questions and my search for the answers are the foundation of this book; its purpose is to open a discussion and shine a light on the explanations and alternative treatments for auto-immune disorders.

Here, we will turn to the realms of vibrational medicine.

For the Western world, the theory behind vibrational medicine (also known as energy medicine) has its initial roots in the early 1900s, and many of its theories and explanations reflect insights that have been discussed in Eastern philoso-phies for millennia. Vibrational medicine sees a human being as a complex network of energy fields that interface with physiology at a cellular level. Vibrational medicine works with specific energies to balance this energetic system when disease has disturbed its equilibrium. To rebalance these energy fields, that will in turn regulate cellular physiology, vibra-tional healers work on restoring harmony in higher levels of human function.

To better understand health from this perspective, we need to address the physical, emotional, mental and spiritual parts of our being. Vibrational medicine and healing consider all these parts and their corresponding vibrations as making up the whole person. Therefore, it is the role of a holistic health practitioner to help restore the coordination and communication between the parts of the whole. Good health is the state of being whole and feeling that all the parts of self are vibrating in concert. This book is designed to assist in the search for that state of health and wholeness.

From time to time I will use case studies from my clinical practice as examples of various conditions and circumstances; of course, the names have been changed. Here are three such cases.

A number of years ago, a young woman came into my clinic complaining of muscle pain, depression, fatigue and problems sleeping. Sabina was one in a long line of similar cases that continue to visit my clinic for relief.

Sabina

Sabina had always enjoyed good health. She worked part-time in her family's busy Italian restaurant, studied music at university, took voice classes and had a small role in an opera. Sabina loved to sing and was sure it was her destiny to become a great opera singer. She was prepared to make whatever sacrifices were demanded. She first came to me thinking she had a bad bout of flu and, since I had helped other members of her family, she wanted the right herbs to make her well again. Sabina was determined to get back to her busy life and, more importantly, the stage.

My initial examination did not indicate flu, and I suggested to her that she needed some relaxing herbs with a tonic action and, at least, a one-month vacation. This was not what she wanted to hear, so she took neither the herbs nor the much-needed rest. Six months later she came to see me again, this time with a diagnosis from her MD of chronic fatigue syndrome and fibromyalgia. Could I fix her?

I started her on a program that consisted of reishi extract, chlorella, beta-carotene, vitamin C and St. John's wort and a whole-food diet that eliminated refined fats, sugars and flours. Since chronic fatigue and fibromyalgia are often associated with particular personality traits, I suggested she also investigate psychological counseling and begin writing a daily journal. Motivated by the constant muscle pain and fatigue, Sabina was now willing to reflect on her physical and emotional habits. Six months later she was not only on her feet, but was auditioning for new singing roles. Within one year, she was back on the stage. Five years later, Sabina was married with one child and another on the way. She is happy taking small parts in the opera until her children are a little older.

Raylin

Raylin was a handsome, highly intelligent fourteen-year-old boy, with a strong body, who suffered from severe asthma. He was a good athlete and loved hockey, but was hampered in competition by not knowing when or if his asthma would prevent him from playing his part at a crucial time in the game. Could I help him? His team and his social life depended on it. He found it devastating to start wheezing with an attack just when the team needed him most. Often, during an intense skirmish on the ice he would suddenly feel his lungs begin to fail. No matter how hard he tried he was unable to get enough oxygen, and the resulting feeling of suffocation scared him. He wanted to know if this was because he was weak. After examining him I assured him he was not weak. In fact, strange though it might seem, his own strength was causing the problem. A weaker body might not have the same type of problem. This sounds like a dichotomy, but because of his own strength, he could store more tension than many others. This tension was then transferred to both his muscles and immune system. The muscles of his chest and bronchial tubes tightened, and his response to the stress acti-vated an immune attack, causing the allergic side of the asthma. I not only had to give him herbal remedies for his condition, I had to understand the psychosomatic dimension of his asthma. Raylin had to learn how to get in touch with his own fears and feelings if he wanted to reduce the asthma attacks.

It took only a few months of daily reishi mushroom supplements (two capsules, twice daily) and a few vitamins for Raylin's asthma attacks to cease. He was back playing on the team but, more importantly, he had learned what most often triggered his attacks. Raylin is feeling much calmer these days, as he has worked out ways to release the tension before it builds up to a critical level. Who knows what he will go on to accomplish.

Maria

Maria suffered with debilitating rheumatic arthritis (RA). She had a hard time walking more than a block without pain. Her hands ached when she tried to make the fresh pasta that she and her husband enjoyed so much. She was also sixty pounds overweight, but could not exercise because of her arthritis. What was she to do? Maria had a strong body and was also quite emotionally sensitive. After discussing her personal life, it was easy to see that she tended to hide her emotions behind a rigid point of view, in order to protect her sensitivity. Besides working on the mechanics of arthritis, she would also have to learn to calm down, and not take everything so seriously: she needed a more flexible outlook.

Maria's body seemed to be attacking her. It took almost one year, but after completing a series of cleanses, using herbal and nutritional supplements, and eventually some regular exercise, Maria's arthritis was gone. She had also lost forty-five pounds. Gradually, she also broadened her perspective, becoming more adaptable. At first these changes came about through her new diet; however, as much of her stress was released, change expanded into other areas of her life.

What do these patients have in common? In each case, the patient had an exceptionally strong body that, it appeared, had turned against itself, resulting in a type of autoimmune disorder. In other words, the immune system launched an attack on its own body, thereby interrupting daily lives, and making it impossible to function normally. How did I help the patients turn things around? Well, in Sabina's case I didn't have a clue, as that was early on in my learning process. I stumbled across a solution without even knowing it. By the time I came to the other cases I definitely had more solid protocols or health programs.

By the time Raylin and Maria came to see me, I knew which key elements would help direct them back to their true healthy selves. These cases and many others helped me fine-tune treatment programs. How did I find these protocols? The answers came after several years of wandering down various treatment paths, many of them therapeutic dead ends, to understand these disorders and to arrive at the various programs—some of which are presented at the end of this book. In the end the answer was clear and simple. It was a matter of creating body harmony by increasing free-flowing communication between various parts of a person's life to stop the stagnation of energy.

A number of common factors underlie many types of autoimmune conditions. In this book, we examine some of these factors, while looking at botanical medicines and other modalities that can help in the management of such conditions.

If we use the traditional metaphor and liken our immune system to an army, most of my patients with autoimmune disorders actually have a stronger than average army on standby. How can we give a strong immune army respect and the power to protect without letting it overtake the body in a coup? This coup is an autoimmune response: the body attacking itself. Can the health and functioning of our immune system be a reflection of the quality of our social interactions? Is the immune system like a tuning fork (a resonator) that reflects the harmonics of the way we perceive our environment? Be ready for some controversy as we look at health and the immune system in a different way.

After observing and working with people in clinical practice for more than thirty years, I find that certain people often end up with autoimmune issues. Most are highly sensitive with no release mechanism for their sensitivity, and are blessed with an exceptionally strong physical constitution. While it may seem strange to claim that those with the strongest bodies often get the worst diseases, with autoimmune disorders this is often the case. Understanding this seeming contradiction was the piece to the puzzle that took me a while to find, and it was only by looking at health beyond the physical dimensions of a disorder that I found the answer.

PART ONE

Autoimmune Diseases

CHAPTER ONE

The Pattern of Emotional Sensitivity

Christina

I entered the clinic waiting room and called Christina. As I glanced over the faces, I quickly double-checked the name on the file. When I said her name, she stood and I scanned her energy. How could this woman be the same Christina? I had not seen her for five years, but she had changed so much I almost failed to recognize her. She had moved to accept a good job out east and her records had gone into our inactive files. I struggled to conceal my surprise at her appearance. She used to have a bounce in her walk, a vivacious smile and almost a glow when she greeted someone. Now, her head was down, she dragged her feet as she slowly crossed the room, and I noticed a gray pallor to her skin.

In the treatment room her story unfolded. Christina's job in the Toronto law firm was good, but demanding. During her first big case, long hours had turned into ridiculous hours; her marriage was on shaky ground; and she had experienced personality conflicts at work. After her first big case she had taken a little time off and recovered to a fair degree. However, the next case was even tougher, especially since she had to work closely with two of the people with whom she had previously been in conflict. Her energy started draining. Now, the few days off between cases barely made any difference to her constant fatigue. However, she kept on working, driven by a substantial mortgage and a new car loan. Within a year she had chronic muscular pain. Hoping it would all go away when the work load lightened, she pushed on. But the fatigue only increased.

After a thorough examination by her MD, she was told that while all of her tests had come back fine, she had chronic fatigue syndrome and fibromyalgia. He offered no solution for these disorders and suggested a long holiday. A holiday was out of the question if she wanted to make partner in the firm, so she kept on working. Six months later, she could not even get out of bed. Thinking she had the flu, she took a day off. A few days turned into a week, and a month later she was no better. Dragging herself back to the doctor's office, she learned that some patients were still dealing with extreme fatigue after four years.

Christina and her husband moved back to Calgary, where she had a better support system of family and friends. Now, even the thought of going back into a law office gave her nightmares. So, here she was back in my clinic. Could I do anything to help her?

Well, I had heard similar stories before. I examined her and, true to her charts, she was really above average health, with an extremely strong constitution. Her immune system seemed to be simultaneously both over- and underfunctioning. Her autonomic nervous system (which maintains many of the body's involuntary functions, such as breathing and digestion) was definitely enervated (overstimulated). To be blunt, she seemed to be living almost exclusively in her head. Despite her illness, she seemed disconnected from her own emotional experiences. I explained that her strong body was actually fighting against her. Her life was like a pressure cooker, with no release valve. Consequently, while she needed to get in touch with her emotional life, her body and mind needed calming. Simple physical activities with a nutritional program became her therapy. I recommended that she start knitting on a daily basis. (I had already observed how the repetitive and rhythmic action of knitting was therapeutic. It seemed to have something to do with the repetitive movements of the hands, and it didn't require strict concentration to be helpful.) The herbal formulas I put her on included reishi, Siberian ginseng, chlorella and some antioxidant vitamins. Then I told her to come back in two weeks.

The process took almost a year before Christina regained her health. However, she still was not well enough to work because every once in a while she seemed to "freeze up" and we would be almost back to zero. The climb back to health was usually much faster. At first I found it difficult to understand what caused these relapses. On the surface, simple stresses often seemed to be involved. Little things (such as the neighbor's cat coming into their yard or her brother tracking dirt into her kitchen) that most people could easily cope with would send her off and she'd be back in bed again. On the other hand, major stress factors, such as their financial difficulties, seemed to have little negative affect. In Christina's transformed state, her coping skills had changed. I remembered those transformer toys my kids used to play with years ago. With just a click, the transformer changed from a person into a war machine. Christina had transformed into a new version of herself. Now it was my job to help her transform back.

George

George was forty-five years old and in good shape but had no idea, until he went for his physical checkup, that he had high blood pressure. His blood pressure was 180 over 110—normal figures for a man his age should be about 130 over 85. The doctor gave him a prescription and sent him home. George was reluctant to take the prescribed drugs and came to me hoping there were herbs he could take instead. I examined George and found him in excellent shape. He was suffering a little from stress, especially his autonomic nervous system, but that seemed minor. I gave him a few simple herbs: garlic, reishi and cayenne and told him to take his own blood pressure every day for a few months. George kept reliable records and we learned that there were minor variations in his blood pressure readings. Stressful events seemed to raise his blood pressure a little, but mostly within an acceptable range—apparently the herbs were working. Two months later George came back. His blood pressure had seemed normal all month long, but when he went to his MD for a follow-up, it registered high again. He got the doctor to take the test twice with different blood pressure cuffs, thinking that there was something wrong with the first one. It was now high again when he came into my office and he wanted to know why the herbs had stopped working. I told him that the herbs could aid his body in fixing the problem, but his problem was also caused by how he interpreted stress. The mere act of being tested would send his blood pressure higher. This particular stress phenomena is called "white coat syndrome."

Cindy

Thirty-six-year-old Cindy came to my office with a diagnosis of irritable bowel syndrome (IBS). She had been referred by her doctor, who had no solution for IBS and had seen many of my patients recover on a herbal and nutritional protocol. After examining her, I found that her overall health was excellent. She worked hard and enjoyed a full life. Everything was fine except for the constant diarrhea, followed by weeks of constipation. She was now in a constipated stage, not having had more than two bowel movements a week for three weeks. She felt bloated and some of her clothes no longer fit. I put her on a herbal detoxification program and started on the process of changing her intestinal tone and normalizing the ecological balance of internal bacteria. She was doing fine for about six months until her daughter came home with a bad report card. The IBS started acting up again. She asked how something as simple as her daughter's report card could set off her IBS, when everything seemed to be going so well?

Stress, sensitivity and autoimmune issues

These three cases all have stress in common. Christina and Cindy are clear cases of autoimmune issues, but George's high blood pressure is not an autoimmune disorder in the traditional sense. However, after many years of clinical practice, I have broadened my definition of autoimmune disorders to include any health condition that appears to be triggered or exacerbated by self-induced stress (as opposed to stress clearly posed by the external environment). Emotional stress seems to be the type of stress that most affects people with autoimmune problems. Oddly, these health problems happen more frequently in my sensitive but genetically or constitutionally strong patients. The pattern I have discovered repeatedly involves stress, sensitivity and auto-immune health.

I had known for a long time that some of my strongest patients were more sensitive, almost intuitive. Often the stronger the constitution, the stronger the intuition. My clinic started to fill with people who had been healthy for most of their lives, but were now coming in with all kinds of serious problems, such as multiple sclerosis, chronic fatigue syndrome and fibromyalgia. Even the younger ones seemed far more susceptible to allergies and asthma or showed signs of attention-deficit disorder (ADD) and attention-deficit hyperactivity disorder (ADHD).

Emotional stress affected these people more than other types of stress, transforming them into some other, almost unrecognizable form of themselves. And the new version didn't include their original strength and ability to adapt to life. They still had the constitutional strength, but they seemed to be stuck in an auto-destruct mode. Their whole energy seemed to be stagnated.

The stress factor

Stress, as a factor in our lives, is not easy to assess. Emotional, mental and physiological stress affect us all differently. In hunter/gatherer societies (more than 95 percent of our history on this planet), stress involved the "fight or flight" response, whereas today our systems seem to be under constant, low-grade stress. The body's stress response is continually turned "on" with occasional crescendos during extra-stressful times. While small amounts of stress are not a bad thing and are a necessary part of life—with the chemical "high" bringing pleasure (thus the enjoyment of roller-coasters, etc.)—long-term, low-grade stress adversely affects the body's systems. Stress has been shown to decrease the functional response of our immune system, thereby reducing resistance to viruses and parasites and creating deficiencies in the immune system.

Different situations cause stress responses in different people. For the group we examine in this book, such stresses are more about the emotional coloration of their lives, which involves people and communication problems. When this group gets into stress-related situations, they do not react with the same fight or flight response as others. Rather, they respond more on an emotional level with symptoms of depression or withdrawal into a closer, group-oriented, support situation.

Such emotionally sensitive people have better nonverbal communication radar than others. For some, the nonverbal (nonlinear) communication cues overshadow verbal (linear) information. Consequently, instead of recognizing the emotional material as someone else's and discarding it or creating a separation from it, the emotional information is kept inside. Internalizing nonlinear data (emotions) and trying to hide behind analytical (linear) explanations will often create circular arguments—made in an attempt to resolve the resulting mental conflict. Sleep is disturbed by going over the event again and again, which in turn creates extra energy that stagnates because the person has not learned how to release it.

Circular arguments become like background noise in the psyche that produces low-grade stress. The combination of stress and circular thinking will often cause many of the body's muscles to tighten, which can affect the tubes of the body, resulting in problems of the digestive tract (poor digestion and constipation;

Crohn's disease or irritable bowel syndrome); respiratory tract illness (allergies, asthma); circulation disorders (high blood pressure); and pain in muscle bundles (fibromyalgia), to mention a few of the most common autoimmune and autoimmune-like disorders.

While some of the emotions we absorb, like love, friendship and the giggles of children playing, are nutritious to our souls, others are not—we will call these emotional roughage. Exactly as food roughage, when eliminated properly, cleanses the gastro-intestinal (GI) tract, so too can emotional roughage cleanse the spirit, if eliminated properly.

This equation explains one of the most basic of natural healing concepts: IN—DO—OUT. In other words, physically, we are what we put into the body, what we do with it and what we do not eliminate. The same is true of the emotional "food" we accept into ourselves. Living with constant emotional background noise and accumulated stress affects the communication systems of our entire body and encourages immune malfunctions. To become truly in touch with our self and return to health, we need to learn how to process all this background noise.

In order to rediscover health and help unravel the mystery of how a healthy person can develop a dramatic autoimmune issue, I am convinced that it is necessary to address the physical, emotional, mental and spiritual dimensions of our being.

Sensitivity and qi stagnation

Christina, who had gone off to Toronto to work as a lawyer, came back almost collapsed with chronic fatigue syndrome and fibro-myalgia. I had been treating Christina and her family since she was six years old. She had always been strong and ambitious, and excelled in school. Christina would definitely be considered a sensitive type. Her sensitivity, combined with her constitutional strength, was now at the root of her health issue.

In a society and culture that emphasizes goal-oriented and task-based behavior, individuals who are more process-oriented and sensitive to emotional information may experience difficulty fitting in. Highly sensitive people pick up more nonlinear data than others and can walk into a room and sense the presence of an argument without having heard anything. Nonlinear data refers to nonverbal communication, such as the body language and positions of people in a room, the emotional ambience in an environment or the tone of a speaker, etc. Some people excel at recognizing and absorbing nonlinear communication. However, if they do not at the same time have suitable release mechanisms for this constant input, they continually build up tension. I see many such patients whose accumulated tension has caused energy stagnation, or what the Chinese would call "qi stagnation." Qi (pronounced "chee" and often written "chi") stagnation breeds disease. This stagnant energy "feeds" microorganisms and may produce any number of health issues, including cysts and tumors.

The old computer saying "garbage in, garbage out" (GIGO) comes to mind. Sensitive individuals simultaneously pick up both healthy and unhealthy emotions from their environment and, in fact, absorb far more emotional information than most individuals. As an analogy (using arbitrary numbers for simplicity), if the average person takes in 100 units of communications a day, these sensitive types pick up at least 200 units a day. Not only are they highly efficient at picking up nonverbal communication, they absorb detail and nuance that most of us miss. While under certain circumstances such receptivity could be considered an advantage, if the sensitivity is hidden (as a social strategy) an imbalance is created. When they take in 200 units, but only release 75 to 100 to the environment, they are internalizing 100 to 125 units a day. At first it might appear that the sensitivity is the problem, but that is not the case.

Most of my patients who developed these health problems also exhibited perfectionist tendencies, and were usually high achievers. Most appeared to be successful in their lives and had worked hard to develop a career, professional title and material prosperity. At least that is how it seemed on the surface. Christina had maintained a perfect grade-point average throughout her academic career and went immediately into practice after graduating. I had never known her to express indecision, confusion or ask others for advice or support. Christina was a perfectionist and she had achieved more than most women her age in a relatively short time, but at what cost?

I have found that the creation of a simple analogy helps me see the question in a different and often simpler light. I knew that I needed to find a model for emotional sensitivity.

Emotional roughage

Absorbing emotions from our environment is similar to eating food. These patients were consuming or extracting more emotions from their environment than the average person. We eat food for many reasons: sometimes for pleasure, because the food looks and tastes good, but on the whole because we need to extract the nutrient value in order to build our physical body. The muscles, glands, organs and brain need to be fed proteins, carbohydrates and sugars to function and stay healthy. However, some of our food has no nutritional value and cannot be digested. We call that roughage: and it is good for us. When a person consumes emotions, the same holds true. Some emotions are nutritious for the soul, while others have no nutritional value. The emotional sensitives were taking in more emotional roughage than the average person; however, roughage was not the problem.

When roughage is held in the digestive tract, this condition is called constipation, which causes all kinds of health problems. Emotional roughage is no different; in other words, many of my patients were emotionally constipated. Christina was certainly holding in a great deal of emotional tension. Our objective was not to lower her sensitivity but to increase her output or expression. After all, consumption without elimination causes a qi stagnation that in turn, no matter where it is located, breeds disease. Regardless of whether the constipation is physical or emotional the result is energy stagnation.

The goal for me was to figure out what caused these patients to change. What was the pressure that triggered the shift from a healthy, active life to an emotionally needy, exhausted existence? To find the answers, I first had to identify which emotions were associated with this imbalance. Any emotion that is picked up from the environment that has no nutritious use for the receiving individual can be considered emotional roughage. This could be simple emotional confusion picked up from another person or very specific emotions that had no application for the individual absorbing them. Such emotional roughage can, and usually does, stimulate emotions within those absorbing them.

The more sensitive a person is, the more emotional roughage he or she will pick up. That is a given. The key is to diffuse the background noise of emotional tension. The most common strategy I see is people wanting to correct this imbalance by blaming their own sensitivity. Instead of learning to process all this emotional data, they try to shut it down or weaken or ignore it. That is a bad plan, because sensitivity is often this person's strongest attribute. Instead of attempting to anesthetize, the policy should be to incorporate a release mechanism into his or her lifestyle.

People who are suffering with these types of autoimmune problems often hide their emotions behind an intellectual or analytical barrier as if they hoped the intellectual veil would keep the world from knowing how sensitive they were. The goal seems to be to have a good "poker face." I began to understand how many of my clients did not want others to know how sensitive they were, so they hid the fact by erecting these intellectual barriers. While this was effective in social situations, what emotional and physical compromises were resulting from the strategy? It seemed that they were just burying the emotional tension even deeper, often even from themselves. There is nothing wrong with this social strategy for people living in our modern day, but they need a release mechanism.

Many of my patients have developed simple release mechanisms for their emotional sponginess, such as keeping a journal, doodling or pounding a drum. Creativity is the best release mechanism for sensitivity. Some people can balance the need to contain their sensitivity (as good social strategy) with the ability to release tension buildup over the weeks, months or years.

Unfortunately, those who could cope were the exception, not the rule. On closer analysis, I noticed that patients who developed autoimmune issues were often living only in their heads. They were disconnected from the body, almost cut off at the neck. Worry, tension, stress and emotional crisis occupied their minds and yet they seemed oblivious to the reality that their being was depositing this stress in the physical body. I looked more closely at their qi patterns—using pulse, tongue and other Oriental diagnostic techniques. It seemed that most of their vital forces had moved more into their head, leaving their energy field barely connected to the body. These patients could articulate and verbalize their symptoms and health concerns in lengthy, often long-winded explanations. Nonetheless, I felt the absence of any passion or desire operating in their lives. They intellectualized everything, including their own physical and emotional issues; while they continued to absorb the emotions of others, they somehow lacked any emotional expression of their own.

To help explain this concept, I have used the following story in my clinic for years. Let us say Betty (an emotional sensitive) is visiting her friend, Jane. Betty is sitting at the kitchen table, while Jane is finishing up the dishes. They are carrying on a conversation. Jane decides to take out the garbage. When she gets outside to the garbage can, she notices that a dog has come along and spread garbage all over the back alley. Of course, Jane is pissed right off. She cleans up the mess, cursing and cussing the whole time. Betty doesn't know anything about this, as she is still in the house. When Jane gets into the house she goes over to the sink to wash off her hands. She looks over to Betty and asks a little louder than normal, "Betty, could you please put the toast in the toaster?" Because Betty is right beside the toaster, of course she puts the toast in the toaster, but what Betty hears is, "Betty, put the toast in the toaster." Because Betty is sensitive, she picks up both nonverbal and verbal communication cues, sensing the hostility behind the words and assuming it is personal. She hears the words "Betty," "toast" and "toaster." By far the loudest words she hears, in flashing neon signs is "pissed off," "pissed off," "pissed off." She might try to analyze this information internally in a linear manner: "Boy, is she pissed off. I wonder why she's pissed off. I'm the only one here. She must be pissed off at me. Wait a minute, I didn't do anything wrong. How could she be pissed off at me? But she sure is pissed off. I must have done something wrong. But I didn't…"

Whenever nonlinear (emotional) data is absorbed and a subsequent attempt is made to apply linear thinking, the result can be the creation of circular arguments and questions that continually revolve in the mind. As there are no answers to these questions, sooner or later the attempt is exhausted and the arguments are buried outside consciousness, and often in the muscular or nervous system.

If we go back and look at the situation more closely and slow it down, we see that Jane spoke politely: "Betty, could you *please* put the toast in the toaster." She even used the magic word! The problem is that because Betty is so hypersensitive, she picked up the mood, or the nonlinear feeling of the speaker, more loudly than she picked up the words. Of course, Betty could ask for more input by inquiring what was wrong and Jane might tell her about the dog and the mess. The whole situation would diffuse and they could laugh about the whole thing. With more linear (intellectual) input, there is no reason for circular arguments. However, there are many instances when it is either inappropriate to ask for more clarification or you might not want to hear the details of someone's life. Consequently, a more broad-based solution is needed for this problem of the increased stress of circular arguments.

Circular arguments

Circular arguments, if left unchecked, are at least partially responsible for many health issues seen in my clinic. This nonlinear
input, for which we have no apparent need, is the emotional
roughage. The continual circular thinking is what keeps people
living in their head and cut off from the body. Many patients
complain of thinking the same thing over and over again, and
described how these thoughts often keep them awake at night.
Usually, these repetitive thoughts were not substantial worries,
like financial or relationship problems. They were small things;
conversations, interactions and ideas from which they could not
escape. These thoughts repeat themselves just like a song or jingle
which, once heard, keeps on playing—even when all is quiet and
sleep is needed.

Sleep disruption is one of the most common problems associated with chronic fatigue syndrome and fibromyalgia. Even
though these patients were continuously fatigued, they still could
not get a full night's sleep. Consequently, they resorted to pharmaceutical sleeping pills that, while giving temporary relief,
certainly did not resolve the underlying problem nor allow for a
deep natural, restful sleep. Sleep evaded these people, allowing for
fewer dreams. Dreams are one of the normal mechanisms that
aid us in dealing with day-to-day frustrations. Dreaming is known
to have important functions about which we still know little,
other than its ability to discharge and process tensions that accumulate during our waking emotional life. The dream world might
provide enough discharge for the average person, and maybe for
the last several thousand years of human history, but for some
reason these emotionally sensitive people are building up more
than they can release through the dream world. They become so

active during these dreaming "detox" or discharging times that the dreams were waking them up and stimulating the physical brain, so they couldn't get back to sleep no matter how tired they were. I often hear them explain that their brain got turned on somehow while they were sleeping and woke them up. If they could only find the switch, they could turn it off and fall back to sleep.

Stress is certainly a part of these issues. This directed my research into understanding more about what went on in the body, due to stress.

SUMMARY POINTS

1. Some of the healthiest people develop some of the most difficult health issues.
2. Many of these people are emotionally sensitive, with a perfectionist streak.
3. Emotional sensitives absorb so much emotional roughage that they have a hard time eliminating.
4. Emotional roughage comes from any emotion that we internalize and for which we have no emotionally nutritious use.
5. Emotional roughage itself is not the problem. It is the holding in of the emotional roughage that creates problems. This is like being exposed to constant low-grade stress.
6. Chronic low-grade emotional stress creates qi stagnation that can transform people into different versions of themselves.
7. Many people hide their emotional sensitivity behind an analytical mental barrier.

8. Creativity assists in releasing emotional roughage.
9. Some people live too much in their head, dissociating from their emotional life.
10. The dream world can also aid in releasing emotional roughage. Sometimes the dreams are so vivid they wake a person up.
11. Autoimmune disorders appear to be associated with a pattern of chronic emotional stress, extreme sensitivity and the inability to discharge emotional tension.

CHAPTER TWO

Stress: Its Role in Health Changes

✿

Anatomy of stress

How does the perception of stress affect health? First, a personal example of perception.

When I was about fourteen, my family had a small but noisy toy fox terrier named Skippy. One morning, while I was raking leaves, the dog discovered a squirrel and chased it up a tree. Now that it had the squirrel "trapped," Skippy felt that it had to keep up the tension to keep the squirrel treed. What followed was a high-pitched chorus similar to a choked machine gun; something that can only come out of a small dog.

The neighbor across the road was out in his front yard. He started yelling at me, so I went across the street to see what he wanted. He was raised up on his feet and leaned forward a bit, as if being bigger would make him more of an authority. Already he was more then a foot and a half taller than me. He projected his voice in a loud tone as if the volume would give him power. "YOU BETTER DO SOMETHING ABOUT THAT DOG, BEFORE I'M FORCED TO." I looked at his furled eyebrows and stern expression. This guy thought he could scare me with his threatening tone. I realized he was taking the whole thing way too seriously. So I immediately said, "You're right, let's kill the little overgrown rat. I'll hold him down and you knock him over the head with your shovel 'til he's dead."

You could see him deflate, and in a tone that now resembled a whiny child he said, "Well I wasn't thinking of going that far. The poor dog, you shouldn't let it outside and allow it to bark like that."

I think that was the first day I consciously realized that stress was all a matter of perception. For whatever reason, this guy was having a bad day and, peeved at the world in general, he wanted to take it out on me and the dog. Had I played along, he would have power-tripped all over me. Energy hitting resistance equals stress. As soon as there was no resistance, there was nothing for his stress response to counter. The situation deflated in an almost comical way. The anger defused and himself unharmed, Skippy stopped barking and ran into the backyard. I returned to finish up with the raking.

Stress, as we perceive and refer to it today, is a relatively modern phenomena. In newspapers or magazine articles from the 1960s, you will never find the word "stress" in the headlines or the text, whereas now the word is in common usage. We assume that we all share the same meaning of stress and frequently describe conditions of stress: we are "stressed out" or "totally stressed" or that we need to "de-stress." In North America, we battle stress daily. Sometimes it seems, we are even proud of our stress.

As hunter-gatherers, our ancestors had the stress response physically programmed into their physiology as a survival mechanism. What was once designed as a survival tool is now the source of an immeasurable amount of disease and illness claiming millions of lives annually. Many holisitic practitioners from various disciplines have estimated that 70 percent to 80 percent of all disease is stress related. At the turn of the twentieth century, the leading causes of death in North America were infectious diseases: influenza, pneumonia, tuberculosis and gastroenteritis. Today, the major causes of death are lifestyle related: coronary heart disease, cancer, stroke and chronic obstructive pulmonary disease. All these diseases have dramatically increased, while at the same time we have more creature comforts and technological gadgets to improve and enhance our standard of living than ever before.

For some there is less money and, for most, less time and more stress. Hand in hand with stress is often an unhealthy lifestyle as people try to "save time" by eating too much fast food and ignoring the need for exercise. Consequently, instead of infectious diseases that can be fought mechanically and chemically, many diseases develop silently over several years or perhaps decades. Today, more than $300 billion a year is spent on lifestyle and stress-related diseases in America. While life expectancy has significantly increased since the turn of the twentieth century, we are now living with disorders and diseases that were almost unknown in the past. Disorders such as chronic fatigue syndrome, syndrome X and fibromyalgia in themselves are on the rise and were unheard of thirty years ago.

Stress: meanings and perceptions

The word "stress," familiar in physics as a description of the tension placed on a physical object, was applied in the human context by Dr. Hans Selye in his classic books *The Stress of Life* and *Stress without Distress*.

In *The Stress of Life*, he described his research into the physiological responses to chronic stress and its relationship with disease (dis-ease). Today, the word is commonly used to describe emotional and mental tensions brought on by the demands of careers, relationships and responsibilities. The average North American now has from 139 to 158 more work hours (annually) than in 1969. Consequently, there is less time for relaxation, the perceived cure for stress. The dividends of the information technology society have proven to be an illusion, as they seem only to result in more stress and significant health deficits.

Depending on an individual's perceptions, stress has many connotations and definitions. In Western culture, stress can be termed as a loss of control; whereas in Eastern cultures, it most often reflects an absence of inner peace. Richard S. Lazarus, noted psychologist and researcher, stated that stress is a state of anxiety produced when events and/or responsibilities exceed one's coping ability. Selye noted that stress is a nonspecific response of the body to cope with and/or adapt to any demand—whether that demand was produced by pleasure or pain. In Chapter 3 I show that both positive and negative experiences produce a physiological stress response, and how the new research from psychoneuro-immunology indicates that the physiological outcome of each can be quite different.

A more holistic definition of stress is a perceived (imagined or real) threat to mental, physical, emotional and spiritual well-being, which results in a response or responses and adaptation. The key word in this statement is "perceived." Take the following example.

A couple win a two-week, all-expenses-paid trip to Hawaii. Most would assume that such an unexpected event would bring both people joy. The wife might start packing immediately, imagining days on the beach, snorkeling along the coral reef and being served drinks by the poolside. On the other hand, the husband is petrified of flying, can't swim, burns too easily and is behind on a deadline at work. The trip would be a complete disaster for him. His stress level goes up even thinking about the win. "Why did she buy that raffle ticket anyway?"

Currently, there is not enough research being done into the effects of emotional stress and what it means to a person's overall health. Most researchers are still back with the physical model: how the physical environment affects the physical body. However, we now know (due to the data from many studies) that perceived emotional or cognitive stressors can be just as real as physical stressors. Both may result in a stress response. The paradigms are a-changing. After all, "shift happens."

Energy view of stress

Another view of stress is as an energy exchange. In other words if stress saps energy, then calmly dealing with change will use less and an anxious response will use more. High-stress situations are exhausting, and this fatigue can become focused in various parts of the body and create symptoms, such as digestive upset, insomnia, fatigue or muscle tension. These symptoms reflect a disruption of energy and thus an interference of the various body systems. Further, stress and anxieties drain the body's energy, which might be needed to work on other health issues.

Both ancient healers from diverse cultures and many contemporary holistic researchers feel that this vital energy is a "gift" from higher realms or what some might call the Great Spirit, God, Goddess or even Mother Nature, or Gaia. In Oriental medicine, the amount of vital energy a person is born with is considered finite. When we exhaust it all, we die. This vital energy can be partially supplemented in several ways. In India they use breathing exercises called Pranayama. Meditation is used to calm down the inner nature, so we use less energy. Nature provides us with vital energy from food, water, air and the awe of its existence. A peaceful walk along a mountain stream among majestic pine trees can do wonders for the soul. The appreciation of a sunset or sunrise has been treasured by many cultures.

From a holistic point of view, it is necessary to understand how the perception of stress as a physical, emotional, mental or spiritual phenomena impacts us.

Stress and the physical body

How does stress affect the physical body? Usually, one of the first answers is Harvard physiologist Walter Cannon's coinage of the phrase the "fight or flight response"—which is the basic response for survival. His research on animals indicated that once a stress was encountered, a response was initiated almost immediately; for example, the fight response was triggered by anger or aggression. Humans also employ the fight response when defending territory or person, which in turn produces physiological preparation for recruiting extra power and strength for short periods of time. We would now call this short, intense anaerobic work. On the other hand, Cannon believed the flight response was caused by fear and was designed to fuel the body to endure prolonged movement, such as running from that proverbial saber-toothed tiger. Fear/flight not only stimulated running, it might also produce behavior such as hiding and withdrawal. This whole fight-flight mechanism is an evolutionary function shared by nearly all of the mammalian species, and is "hardwired" into the human physiology.

While this response mechanism is very effective for managing physical stress or threat, it is a rather antiquated mechanism for coping with many of today's stresses. The fight or flight response has not kept pace with the development of the human mind and socialization. Nowadays, the more common stresses are psychological in nature. The problem is that the same physiological mechanism is initiated, regardless of whether the stress is of a physical or mental nature. The body enters this state of readiness whether there is perceived stress, such as being late for an important meeting, being humiliated or thinking there's a monster under the bed. Cannon noted the physiological actions of the fight or flight response effect almost every physiological system. Here are just a few (see Figure 2.1):

- Increased heart rate to pump blood to working muscles
- Increased blood pressure to deliver blood to working muscles

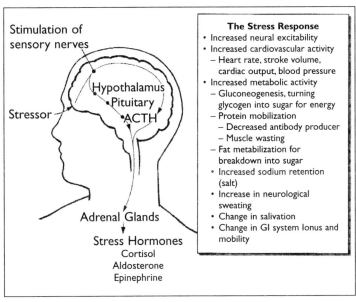

Stimulation of sensory nerves

Hypothalamus
Pituitary
ACTH

Stressor

Adrenal Glands

Stress Hormones
Cortisol
Aldosterone
Epinephrine

The Stress Response
- Increased neural excitability
- Increased cardiovascular activity
  – Heart rate, stroke volume, cardiac output, blood pressure
- Increased metabolic activity
  – Gluconeogenesis, turning glycogen into sugar for energy
  – Protein mobilization
    – Decreased antibody producer
    – Muscle wasting
  – Fat metabilization for breakdown into sugar
- Increased sodium retention (salt)
- Increase in neurological sweating
- Change in salivation
- Change in GI system Ionus and mobility

FIGURE **2.1**

- Increased ventilation to supply working muscle with more oxygen for metabolic energy
- Vasodilation (widening of blood vessels) of arteries to body's periphery (arms and legs) with the greatest muscle mass
- Increased serum glucose for metabolic processes during muscle contraction
- Increased free fatty acid mobilization as an energy source for prolonged activity (e.g., running)
- Increased blood coagulation and decreased clotting time in the event of bleeding
- Increased muscle strength
- Decreased gastric movement and abdominal blood flow to allow blood to go to working muscles
- Increased perspiration to cool body-core temperature

The problem in modern society is that while these responses are efficient for escaping from a physical danger, they are quite ineffective when dealing with an event that threatens to upset our psychological identity, the dilemma being that our body reacts the same way whether the perceived threat is physical, emotional, mental or spiritual in nature. If we are under relatively constant survival threats and unable to return to homeostasis (a steady state in the body's internal environment, maintained by various feed-back and control mechanisms), the result is an extremely negative effect on most of the body's systems, such as the cardiovascular, digestive, musculoskeletal and the immune systems.

Fight or flight revisited

Imagine a group of deer peacefully grazing in a mountain meadow when suddenly one of them sees something moving in the grass. Danger is sensed and the deer are instantly ready for flight. It is nothing, and they continue grazing. At that moment a pack of wolves rushes from the undergrowth, and in one big wave the deer take off.

One of the smaller deer slips for an instant, then recovers, but it is too late—a wolf lunges. At that moment, rigid and apparently lifeless, the young deer falls to the ground uninjured and surrenders to its impending death. The deer is not pretending to be dead, rather it has entered an altered state of consciousness that is shared by all mammals when death seems imminent. Some indigenous people feel this phenomenon is the surrender of the spirit of the prey to the predator, which it could very well be.

This is called "immobility" or the "freezing" response. This is the third state of response available to reptiles and mammals when facing overwhelming threat. The fight or flight model is only part of our current understanding. Freezing is just as important. Many animals freeze in the face of danger. This is an important evolutionary feature that is conserved in the evolutionary chain in all higher mammals, including humans. Our muscles freeze, as if we are playing dead, as a last-ditch survival strategy.

Freezing has many advantages. Playing "possum" will often deter predators. If the victim plays dead it may appear to be "bad meat," or possibly it just takes the fun out of the chase—the cat and mouse idea. In this excited state of altered reality, higher levels of endorphins are produced, and the prey feels little pain. In this way, nature ensures the animal does not have to feel the agony of being torn limb from limb. Thinking the deer is dead, the wolf might drag the deer back to the den to share with its cubs. If the victim has a chance, it can awaken from its frozen state and escape and, once out of danger, will literally shake off the residual body effect and return to its normal life. Humans have similar reactions when facing certain types of stress.

The work of Peter Levine, Ph.D., in his book *Walking the Tiger: Healing Trauma,* shows a completely new view of how humans trap emotional traumas in muscles and viscera. He states that remaining in that "frozen" state results in muscle problems, possibly even problems like fibromyalgia in the long run. To cure the residue from undischarged stress, we have to unlock or thaw the trauma. Freezing occurs when there is no other course of action. The trigger can be as dramatic as a plane crash or a car accident or as simple as the buildup of everyday frustrations. For example: You are standing in front of the photocopier and the boss comes along and starts to make all sorts of intimidating remarks. In a fight or flight response you would either hit him/ her or run out of there. But because your rational nature tells you to stay and be quiet because you need that job, you just bury or freeze the situation into your body.

In her insightful book, *Betrayal, Trust and Forgiveness: A Guide to Emotional Healing and Self-Renewal*, Beth Hedva, Ph.D., introduced more levels and cited movement psychologist (and sixth-degree black belt martial artist) Stuart Heller, Ph.D., who added fainting to the animal and human range of stress responses; stating that the adrenal response is wired through a fear response of faint, fight, flight and freeze. For example:

- The possum will faint to look dead to a predator. For humans, the faint response is one of denying, forgetting or feeling confused.
- When this denial mechanism is challenged anger quickly evolves into the equivalent aggressive fight response of a wolverine.
- The flight response is like a flock of birds that takes to the sky to avoid a predator. In humans, this response often expresses

itself as avoidance, rationalization or running away with an idea to avoid reality.

- Freezing often shows up as sadness, crying and depression. The person might feel stuck, heavy or immobilized by emotions.

Today, we are exposed to continuous faint, fight, flight or freeze situations, often of an emotional nature. Divorce, financial crisis, career changes and relationship conflicts are part of the contemporary landscape. The ensuing stress seldom contains a physical stimulus and therefore has no physical output. When we have time to relax, we might choose excessive exercise (enough to produce an endorphin high) to make us feel temporarily better. However, this may further stress the same tissue that is wearing out due to the overactive fight or flight situation. Consequently, the system remains under constant, low-grade stress, even during "relaxation." Obviously exercise in moderation is a good thing. However, using exercise as an escape, always producing high endorphin levels, is not that different from using drugs to escape and, in addition, can damage tissue.

Neurotransmitters and the molecular dance

How are perceptions of stress communicated within the brain? The smallest functional part of the nervous system is the neuron (see Figure 2.2). Neurons communicate with each other through chemicals called neurotransmitters, which help transfer information from one neuron to another. The first neuron sends out one of these neurotransmitters, which is received by a receptor site on the next neuron across a space called a synapse (see Figure 2.3). These receptor sites are tiny molecules that cover the surface of the neuron. A single neuron can contain millions of receptor sites.

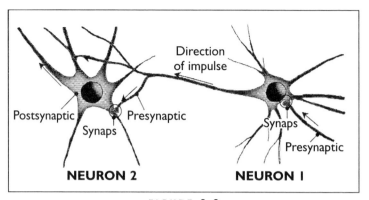

Direction of impulse

Postsynaptic

Presynaptic

Synaps

Synaps

Presynaptic

NEURON 2

NEURON I

FIGURE **2.2**

These receptor sites are now known to be flexible molecules. They can wiggle, shimmy and even hum as they change shapes between two or three favored shapes. The receptor sites float above the surface of a cell's membrane, like lily pads floating on a pond. They receive the information and send it deep into the cell, like the lily's roots, anchoring themselves to the pond floor.

The receptors are like sensing molecules or scanners, acting like eyes, ears and taste buds, but on a cellular level—hovering over the surface of the cell, dancing and vibrating, waiting to meet up with a similar molecule. Both transmitter and receptor molecules are made of amino acids. When the right molecule comes along, they dance with the molecule—like sex on a molecular level. These sexual partners are very selective and will have sex only with a partner that knows the same dance. As soon as it finds the right partner the molecule gets tickled into rearranging itself, changing shape until—click—the information enters the cell. These receptor sites are very specific; for example, an opiate receptor site can receive information only from molecules that

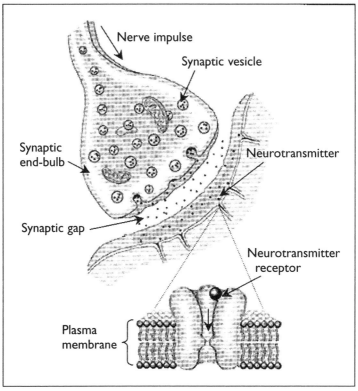

FIGURE **2.3**

have opiate shapes, like morphine, heroin or endorphins. Valium receptor sites can get information only from valium and valium-like molecular shapes.

Endorphins and mood

There is a special category of molecules that needs explanation: the endorphins. This group of communicators and their receptor sites strongly influence our moods. The receptor sites for endorphins are the same ones involved in heroin and opium addiction. In fact, we can say that endorphins are the body's own type of opium: manufactured by the body, they regulate stress, pain, moods, sexuality, appetite, addictions, substance abuse and sports performance. They produce the highs and lows of life, without which it would be boring. Endorphins are also produced by increasing aerobic exercise—the wall or second wind that runners talk about, and the "high" produced by certain types of exercise.

However, these endorphin "rushes" can become addictive. In order to maintain the "high," the ante must be steadily increased: running further, skiing harder, etc. The increased activity level can not only cause physical injury as the person exercises beyond his or her ability; the individual can also become addicted to his or her own personally produced brand of opium: "endorphins." Such addiction can cause additional damage, as the extreme activity exposes the body to constant stress. This is not to say that exercise is bad, but that excessive exercise can cause the very thing we are trying to fix: producing high levels of stress on tissue while ignoring signals from the physical body. This pattern has become apparent in chronic fatigue syndrome patients. Once they began to feel better, they tend to quickly return to their exercise program, only to relapse into a fatigue syndrome. Moderate exercise is good; excessive exercise can cause problems for some people.

During my research on how endorphins operate, I came across the work of one of the discovers of endorphin and their receptors sites, Candice Pert.

Even a biochemist believes the mind is not only in the brain

In the late 1980s and early 1990s, Candace Pert, Ph.D., former Chief of Brain Chemistry at the National Institute for Mental

Health, proved that there were receptor cells for brain neuro-transmitters throughout the body. Until recently there was not thought to be any direct link between the nervous system and the immune system; virtually all physiologists believed that these two systems worked independently. Researchers have now found several neural connections from the central nervous system (CNS) to the thymus, lymph nodes, spleen, bone marrow, tonsils, adenoids and Peyces cells in the small intestine—all part of the immune system.

A second and, perhaps, more significant link is that neuropeptides, produced in the brain, have receptor sites throughout the immune system. Pert and others have shown that these neuropeptides are responsive to emotions—thereby establishing a direct emotional link between the brain and the body's immune system. The endorphins, among at least sixty identified neuropeptides, are associated with mood and immune regulation. Pert has further suggested that there might only be one neuropeptide molecule, which, like a chameleon, changes configuration as a result of emotional influence. Apparently, it is the frequency at which the molecule vibrates that determines its function and relationship to the receptor site. This is important because it fits well with the concept of vibrational medicine and, as we shall see, the electro-magnetic frequency model of cell reception.

At one point, it was believed that these neuropeptides were produced only in the brain; now we know that the immune system can manufacture them in response to emotional stimuli. This confirms a two-way communication system on a physical level between at least these two systems. We now know that part of the immune system, like the T- and B-cells, has a bidirectional pathway of communication between the brain and the central nervous system.

In 1987, Pert stated, "I think it is possible now to conceive of mind and consciousness processing and as such mind and consciousness would appear to be independent from brain and body." There are now many doctors and researchers (e.g., Joan Borysenko, Ph.D., Larry Dossey, MD, Deepak Chopra, MD and Bernie Siegel, MD) looking beyond the physical body to understand the puzzling relationship between stress and disease.

Emotional development and stress

Researchers have found that while certain human functions are found in both sides of the brain, others are located primarily on either the left or right hemisphere. The left is better equipped to process language, linear thought, analysis, logical and serial phenomena. The right is utilized in processing nonverbal activities such as music, spatial and visual information. Since this research emerged it is common to refer to the right brain as artistic, poetic and holistic or more yin; and the left as linear, analytical or more yang.

Most North Americans and Europeans are well trained in processing linear, serial phenomena or left brain tasks—basically the emphasis of our educational system. Aside from some physical education, it unfortunately tends to end there. Most of us are highly illiterate when it comes to processing emotional information, or expressing ourselves emotionally. Many other cultures, especially tribal societies, integrate emotional education into their daily life, which can take the form of story telling, rituals and rites, like coming-of-age ceremonies; such activities are necessary for the survival of tight-knit groups. To become whole, productive members of society, we also need an emotional education. In our society we seem to bypass this process and reward left brain achievements exclusively.

Creative and artistic expression is an integral aspect of human experience and necessary for health and well-being. Input without a proper release again produces stagnated qi. Qi stagnation can cause inflammation and even tumor systems. A useful comparison is stagnant water that creates an environment in which algae, mosquitoes and bacteria breed. Our society rewards people for personal achievements and perfectionism. There is nothing wrong with taking pride in a job well done, and there is certainly room for perfection in a person's life. However, for some, the quest is overpowering. Perfectionism can be overwhelming and all-consuming, which, in turn, will create stagnation. Unfortunately, the more prevalent the perfectionism, the more isolated the individual will feel. One of the more common health problems that I see can be summed up in one word—loneliness. While many perfectionists have huge networks of friends and co-workers, they also feel disconnected and that they are shouldering society, or the universe, all on their own.

In the past, collective social activity was one way we dealt with excess stress and tension. In North America, shared gatherings in public places have been replaced with private activities such as watching a video at home, spending time on the Internet or talking on the telephone. Some of our strongest shared experiences have occurred through the medium of television news broadcasts. We are at once alone and yet part of a collective communicative experience. On the other hand, many societies in India, Asia, and South and Central America still celebrate traditional festivals at least every two to three months. All the shops shut down and the whole society leaves its regular routine to join in the festival for a few days. En masse they celebrate, mourn or go through the emotions of that particular festival. For some festivals, people disguise themselves with costumes, or get inebriated for days, but are able to get back to normal at the end of the festival. In other festivals, people pray collectively, or ask for forgiveness of various spirits. There are as many themes as there are festivals, but when the festival is over, everyone gets back to normal everyday life. Those who were walking around nude a few days earlier are now back in business attire, going about their normal work, running their shops and selling their vegetables. The festival is over, the tension is released and now normal life resumes. Collectively, people have experienced what is known as the "liminal," or an altered reality, during a festival or carnival. This type of release is a function of the right brain. The linear rational everyday world of responsibility is set aside so that we can enter the theater of magic and emotion. The liminal is a place of twilight, between worlds, where color, image, sound and movement express the mysteries of being human. Festivals refresh, rejuvenate and release individual and group tension.

While of course there are various community events and national celebrations in the West, for the most part these do not "engage" or encourage active participation—it would be much healthier for everyone if they did.

We have all experienced the collective "high" created when a group is focused and moving or singing in unison. The crowd's energy produces a dramatic "mind" of its own. The phenomena of a group creates a mass of energy that can be directed in any number of ways. Dramatic examples of this were seen in the mass outpouring of grief after Princess Diana's death and the tragedy of September 11, 2001. We now know a great deal about how tension and stress impact us physically and emotionally; yet the numbers of people with autoimmune disorders exacerbated by stress continues to grow. Some of the most exciting research, such as that done by Candace Pert, also raises questions about the nature of mind and consciousness. In other words, if stress is perceived in the mind, where exactly is that located? While we continue to learn more about the connections between our nervous system, immune system, emotions and well-being, major questions about healing remain unanswered riddles. There are many health-related issues that plainly have no physical or logical explanation. These inexplicable cases lead us to search beyond the physical dimension for enlightenment. The following examples of these unresolved questions may show a pattern.

Unresolved questions in medical literature

Multiple personality disorder (MPD)

It has been shown that people diagnosed with MPD can often manifest different illness with different personalities. For instance, a patient is diabetic in one personality but not in other personalities, or a patient needs prescription glasses in one personality but not in others. How can there be a completely different set of diseases from one personality to the next? What do MPD patients have in common? In their youth, most have experienced some incredibly traumatic event. If, once a person became diabetic from damage, the trauma had effected on the physical body, we would expect he or she to remain diabetic in all personalities. However, apparently some other control mechanism is functioning here. Is there some sort of electromagnetic control or higher-level mechanism either increasing or decreasing energy over an area due to the emotional trauma? How and why is the other personality not being influenced by the same trauma?

Spontaneous Remission

In 1982, I saw Katey, a nineteen-year-old diagnosed with breast cancer. She was an attractive young woman who never wore a bra and was extremely self-conscious about her larger than normal breasts. One of her doctors suggested that not wearing a bra was the most likely cause of her condition. After discussing this with me, she stated that she didn't have nice breasts as they were too large. When she was walking down the street, her breasts would flop around. Many people (especially men) looked at her breasts and she felt this was because they were unattractive. I assured her that many of the people watching her walk down the street were not imagining that they were unattractive.

Katey was about to have a radical mastectomy to remove her left breast—and for some months I had given her supplements to build up her system for the operation. During this time, she met a young man with whom she had a three-day affair. At the end of the weekend, she had discussed with him where their relationship might go from there. He said to her, " Relationship with you? You were the worse lay I've ever had. Why would I want to spend time with you?" One can imagine how this would affect the average person, especially a nineteen-year-old who already had feelings of inadequacy about her sexuality. This made Katey look deep into herself and she came to the conclusion that, in fact, they had both enjoyed lots of fun over the weekend. For whatever reason, her male partner was unable to give her positive acknowlededgement. She felt good about their experience together, except for the final rejection.

Who knows why the man made this statement, but it had a profound effect on her. The next week when she went for her pre-operation examination there was no sign of the cancer. Several tests were done, but somehow she had spontaneously healed. This was the first time I had witnessed such a case. Certainly, I had given her some herbs; however, my sense is that her healing came in that brief moment when she had to readdress her own self-worth and sexuality, and decided that, after all, she was all right.

There are many examples of spontaneous healing in the medical literature and, through the years, I have witnessed several cases. What causes it? A change in the emotional response to the world; therefore a change in the person's emotional world; thus no need for the illness anymore? Typically, the first reaction from hidebound/conservative members of the medical community is denial, with the standard explanation that there was a misdiagnosis in the first place.

In the mid-1980s, the Institute of Noetic Sciences found more than 3,000 cases of spontaneous remission in the medical literature. In 15 percent of the cases nothing was prescribed for the patients, as it was felt their conditions were incurable. There is still no explanation as to why some people can go to "faith healers" and be spontaneously healed. Fifty percent of the people who went to the Shrine of St. Bernadette at Lourdes over a ten-year period and were healed received no medical explanation for their spontaneous healing from the International Medical Commission of Lourdes that investigated them.

Hypnosis can access the unconscious mind and create documented physiological changes that are baffling. Hypnosis has been used to cure addictions, warts, asthma, hay fever, contact dermatitis and other allergies. While hypnosis is known to relax a person and enhances the immune system, this alone cannot account for the major hormonal changes and shift in the disease's symptoms.

Placebos and nocebos have been classified in the area of faith healing. If a person strongly believes in the healing properties of something, it will often have a healing effect. Placebos are inert substances that are given in trials to test the difference between the "active drug" and the inert one. The placebo effect is so strong that the Federal Drug Agency (FDA) insists that new medications must produce a cure rate of more than 35 percent — the demarcation of the placebo effect—in clinical trials before they are approved. Dr. Bernie Siegel, author of the book *Love, Medicine and Miracles*, suggests that the placebo effect more likely explains 70 percent of healing. He gives many examples of how patients were cured or had their lives extended by the attention their health-care provider gave them, rather than from an ingested substance. This type of faith healing is not fully understood, but it does point to a bigger picture. Healing often takes place in the mind or emotions, outside the physical realms of medicine.

Nocebos are the opposite: a substance given to a patient that has been shown to be very effective, but the patient is told that the substance is just part of an experiment that most likely will not work. Here, the medication is found to be ineffective in the presence of belief. Again, we observe the power of mind over matter.

Julia

Throughout the years I have had many cases like Julia's. I first saw her in 1997, when she had a moderately severe case of depression. For years she used prescribed antidepressants but had stopped taking them as she did not like their effects. She had read about the new wonder herb for depression, St. John's wort.

I gave her some tincture and the effect was miraculous; her depression was gone in less than a week. She reported that she felt more like herself than she ever did on the pharmaceuticals like Prozac and Paxil.

Her sense of well-being continued—for at least five months—until her semiannual appointment with her psychiatrist who was appalled that she had ceased taking her medication. Didn't she know that there was no scientific proof for St. John's wort? Nonetheless, she continued using the herb despite her psychiatrist's opinion. About two months later, she came to me again and said that the herb was not working any more, and proceeded to tell me about the incident with her psychiatrist. I gave her a stack of papers of the research done on St. John's wort that I was preparing for my advanced herbal students. Julia took the material home and read it. Two weeks later, in a follow-up visit, she was happy to report that the herb was again working well.

There have been many studies done on St John's wort. In Germany alone there are more than two million prescriptions written annually by medical doctors—about five times the number for Prozac.

Julia's story shows that often treatment can take place outside the realms of physiological explanation. Stress and belief are significant factors in disease. They impact us at the emotional and mental level as much as in the physical body. It is the job of the health care provider to determine where the center of gravity of the health issue is located and proceed to use remedies that will affect that part of the person.

One of the areas most affected by emotional stress is the immune system, especially autoimmune issues.

SUMMARY POINTS

1. Stress is a matter of perception; what is stressful for one might not be for another.

2. Contemporary definitions of stress are relatively new.

3. The word "stress" derives from physics and describes the tension or force placed on an object to bend or break it.

4. In Western culture, stress can be termed as a loss of control. In Eastern cultures, stress can reflect an absence of inner peace. A more holistic definition of stress is a perceived (imagined or real) threat to one's mental, physical, emotional and spiritual well-being, which results in a response, or responses, and adaptation.

5. The fight or flight response to stress was first described in 1914.

6. We have the same physiological response to stress whether the stress is physical or psychological.

7. Our physiological responses to stress are effective for escaping physical dangers but inadequate for dealing with psychological issues.

8. As well as the fight or flight response to stress, we may also faint or freeze.

9. The hemispheres of the brain tend to govern different types of tasks and functions. Left brain functions are more linear, logic-based and sequential; right brain functions are more holistic, creative and nonverbal.

10. North American society tends to exclusively reward and train individuals in left brain processing tasks. When we ignore right brain nonverbal expressive activity in our lives, we may accumulate chronic tension. We call this qi stagnation. Qi stagnation can produce disease.

11. Although science has uncovered much information about how stress impacts our physical and emotional well-being, and how the brain functions, unresolved medical phenomena point to an explanation for, and of, health that goes beyond the purely physical dimension.

Psychoneuroimmunology

❖

Social aspects of stress

The impact on health from many types of social stressors has been the subject of much research, and there is an increasing amount of resulting data suggesting that the emotional stress we perceive in our environment has a direct effect on our health. Further, certain individuals seem to be more affected than others.

This data provides overwhelming evidence of the direct effect of this stress on the immune system. One would expect that the death of a spouse would cause immunosuppression (lowering of the body's normal immune response to the invasion of foreign material/s), but traumatic marital separation has been shown to be more immunosuppressive than bereavement. Low-grade chronic stress, termed "microstress," may be even more immunosuppressive than either death or separation. Major trauma causes stress but the stress of ongoing, day-to-day hassles can also take a strong toll on the immune system. From an evolutionary perspective, we are better suited for the flight or fight response to dramatic stress than to continual low-grade stress. Some studies show that people who perceive themselves to be under continuous stress are more likely to get infections, such as upper respiratory tract infections. Further, chronic stress has been shown to impair healing, while reducing immune system communication. In addition, it appears that emotional "memory" will often enhance the degree to which the stress affects the immune system.

We all have various group memories that have associated emotional charges and that are triggered by many contextual cues. In other words, different social memories are embedded in our being. For example, some people know exactly what they were doing when President Kennedy was shot or when John Lennon died or, more recently, when the twin towers of the World Trade Center were attacked. Contextual cues from these stored memories can create stress and immune responses in the body. We also have our own personal contextual cues related to past incidences and emotional experiences in our life, which trigger both emotional and immune responses.

Major trauma, especially if experienced early in life, can cause problems later in life and contribute to stress responses of which we are not consciously aware. Known as post-trauma syndrome (PTS), unresolved trauma can highjack the nervous and immune system, triggering health issues in what seem to be mysterious ways. Originally, PTS was thought to affect only the survivors of war or severe trauma on that scale, however, in recent years the category has been expanded to include emotional stresses, such as abuse and neglect. For a practitioner trying to help a patient regain his or her health, PTS is one of the most stubborn blocks to break down. These blocks, created from unresolved trauma, need to be deprogrammed or unlearned, as they were behaviorally programmed in the first place. A simple example from animal research illustrates this. An aversion experiment was set up by Dr. R. Alder in 1975, wherein he taught rats to avoid sugar water by simultaneously administering cyclophosphamide, a tasteless nonimmunosuppressive drug that induces nausea. Later, when the rats were reintroduced to the sugar water without the cyclophosphamide, they still developed nausea, which was not unexpected. However, the rats then started to die of infections, and it was shown that the sugar water had had a powerful immunosuppressive effect. Under normal stress-free conditions, sugar water would not suppress the animals' immunity to this degree. There was considerable skepticism about this study, when it was suggested that the immune system could be classically conditioned in the same way as behavior and physiological responses. Since then, these results have been extensively replicated and studied, and it is now known that animals can learn to suppress or enhance the function of many parts of the immune system (T-cells, B-cells, cytotoxic cells, NK-cells and mast cells).

This fact, and other evidence, has shown that psychosocial disruption that occurs in the womb, after birth and during childhood, can have long-term consequences for the immune system. Thus, trauma experienced in youth may result in poorer coping responses to stress in adulthood—by which time strategies for coping with stress have been shown to be important in terms of how stress will affect the immune system. There have been several studies with acute asthma attacks, viral infection, AIDS, cancer and heart disease suggesting that stress-coping strategies can minimize or enhance the duration and/or degree of the health issue.

This is not to say that we are all irreversibly programmed in the womb or as children. New coping strategies can be learned. For the most part, how we cope with stress, at any age, is a learned skill. Sometimes we have to unlearn poor coping responses, such as substance abuse, and learn new ways to deal with stress. New traumas may also occur. There is sufficient evidence to suggest that social support, which encourages the cognitive handling of emotionally charged information, can impact mortality, further reinforcing the position that the immune system can no longer be considered as a separate player in our body. Virtually every aspect of immune function influences the nervous system and their neuropeptides, which in turn, affect the immune system in a two-way flow of information, exchanging and regulating each other. This highlights two major facts:

1. The breakdown in cooperation between the communication system inside the body may underlie many diseases. Stress and/or trauma may precipitate this breakdown.

2. By medicating only one part of the system and ignoring other parts, the whole system may be thrown into chaos, thereby aggravating the health issue. For example, prescribing only Prozac to reduce depression will change the function and levels of serotonin (a chemical widely distributed in the body, especially in the brain where it acts as a neurotransmitter) and thus dramatically affect the immune system, which will in turn feed back more information to the nervous system, creating a vicious spiral of health decline. Prozac use can affect immune function.

One of the new research areas, in the field of integrated health, goes by the jaw-breaking name psychoneuroimmunoen-docrinology. It is the study of how the emotional, neurological, immunological and endocrine systems interrelate in one large communication system. This has been popularized and the word shortened (only a little!) to become psychoneuroimmunology (PNI). We now know that stress can weaken or damage the immune system, and PNI examines the interaction and relationships between immune functioning and behavior. Immune responses to stress, which affect our mood and behaviors, are mediated by the nervous system. When we think about the influence of stress on our health, we must consider the immune and nervous systems as well as our psychological makeup. This field of study is proving that many health issues are made up of three distinct parts:

1. Psychological
2. Neurological
3. Immunological

The root of a health issue may vary from person to person albeit with the same health diagnosis or set of symptoms, and may occasionally vary within the same person. For example, chronic fatigue syndrome is a clear example of a disease with immune, neurological and psychological elements. For this reason, it is often difficult to diagnose as the symptoms might appear more psychological in one person and more immune-based in another, and the symptoms can also change over time for an individual. While this is challenging for the health care practitioner, for researchers it is an exciting field that is yielding knowledge about the complex interconnections between disease and well-being.

A practitioner who employs PNI theory has to combine an understanding of neurochemicals with knowledge of immune, endocrine, neural and psychological functioning. As well, the implications and potential for cross-talk between the endocrine, immune and nervous systems are studied. PNI research now encompasses diseases that include autoimmune, neurological and psychiatric issues. The harmony and imbalance of the immune, endocrine and neurotransmitter systems and their resulting relationships is also being studied. Even though this line of research has turned many schools and medical practices almost upside down, it has provided a rationale for validating some psychosomatic diseases, like chronic fatigue syndrome or many of the social-psychological aspects of rheumatoid arthritis and systemic lupus erythematosus (SLE) that have been marginalized for decades.

Even though PNI researchers and practitioners have provided convincing evidence for a greater degree of functional integration between systems of the body, this is not to say they have all embraced the concepts of vital energy. In fact, most have not; however, it is intriguing to see that many are. To hear senior neurologists or endocrinologists talking about meditation, tai chi and energy flow is encouraging.

An interconnected view of the immune and nervous systems, which includes behavior and the role of stress in health and disease, is a great departure from the basis of most Western medical theory since the time of René Descartes, the seventeenth-century French philosopher and mathematician. Descartes proposed that the complex study of living organisms could best be understood by investigating the individual components that comprised the individual. His idea assumed that by studying smaller and smaller component parts of the body it would be easier to understand how the whole worked.

Descartes was a curious combination of materialist, dualist and metaphysician. Although he acknowledged the existence of a God, his reasoning resulted in the notion that the natural and physical worlds were entirely separate from those of the mind and the divine. His universe was a mechanical one in which material and physical things were governed by only natural causes and natural effects. The mind, however, was entirely separate and not subject to the same natural laws as the body. Reductionism, the scientific theory that all biological processes are governed by the same laws of chemistry and physics, is traceable to the reasoning of Descartes and the subsequent popularization of his ideas. By the nineteenth century, body and mind had become completely separate disciplines; the study of mind and soul belonged to the theologians and philosophers, and the body to the world of the physiologist, anatomist and clinicians. This has influenced medical theory to this day. But what Descartes also made possible, in his separation of the mind from the body, was the eventual birth of psychology as its own discipline. Today, we now have a wealth of knowledge and research in the area of PNI, and after you get through all the jargon and complicated pathways it almost reads like a page out of a holistic practitioner's manual. Without a shadow of a doubt, it has been proven that what is felt in the emotions can influence the immune system. In the clinical situation, we see this all the time.

Autoimmunity

When a person's immune system turns against itself, we say the person has developed an autoimmune disorder. The autoimmune health disorders appear to be particularly linked to stress and the ability to successfully cope with social and emotional stressors. The most common autoimmune diseases are:

- Multiple sclerosis (MS)
- Type 1 (juvenile) diabetes
- Rheumatoid arthritis
- Vitiligo (patches of skin lacking pigment)

- Thyroid inflammation (Hashimoto's or Graves' disease)
- Systemic lupus erythematosus (SLE)
- Inflammatory bowel disease (IBS, Crohn's disease or ulcerative colitis)
- Myasthenia gravis (muscle weakness)
- Liver inflammation (primary biliary cirrhosis or chronic active hepatitis)
- Destruction of blood platelets (idiopathic thrombocytopenic purpura (ITP))
- Eye inflammation (uveitis)
- Kidney inflammation (glomerulonephritis)
- Scleroderma (unneccessary scar tissue formed in skin and other organs)
- Pemphigus (blisters of the skin)

In addition to these classical autoimmune diseases that are direct attacks of the immune system on the body, I use a more liberal definition of autoimmune disorder which includes any attack of the self against itself (may it be immune, neural, endocrine or even psychological), such as:

- Allergies (often considered in the first list)
- Asthma
- Chronic fatigue syndrome
- Fibromyalgia
- Many forms of cancer
- Certain types of high blood pressure
- Syndrome X (a new term for a number of conditions that, when occurring simultaneously, may indicate a predisposition to diabetes, heart disease and a large number of other problems)

Many of these diseases are due to enervation of the autonomic nervous system. While these disorders are not classic autoimmune disorders, they are definitely PNI issues. In other words, the immune system is being compromised by a combination of psychological and nervous system factors. This broader definition emerges out of dysregulation of any part of the body-mind that attacks itself. The result may produce an aspect of inappropriate healing, as well as tissue destruction that leads to further disease. This type of autoimmune malfunction is an undesirable force with a damaging pattern of reaction. These malfunctions are caused by conflicts in signals influenced by genetic predisposition or immune, nervous, psychological or vital energy factors feeding back to the self.

There is no doubt that there are some genetic aspects to certain autoimmune issues. The areas are well studied for genetic predispositions associated with type 1 diabetes, multiple sclerosis, Hashimoto's disease and other classical autoimmune issues. These predispositions or susceptibilities are just that, not causes. Most people with these genetic predispositions will never develop the related issue. Monozygotic (or identical) twins develop from a single fertilized egg cell, thus inheriting the same set of genes. If one twin develops type 1 diabetes or rheumatoid arthritis, that does not mean the other will. In fact, it is rare that twins would share an autoimmune issue. Even identical twins deal with their environment individually and develop different coping styles or learn different skills. It appears that it takes some outside environmental factor to turn on the genetic potential.

Gender and autoimmune diseases

Another pattern that might seem genetic at first is gender. In the world of autoimmune disease a very marked, but perplexing, observation can be made. Women tend to develop far more auto-immune issues than men. Initially, researchers believed this was related to the X and Y chromosome, but this proved not to be the case. Nonetheless, a pattern exists. Systemic lupus erythematosus (SLE) is ten times more prevalent in women; Graves' disease of the thyroid is seven times higher; while rheumatoid arthritis and myasthenia gravis are three times higher. Eighty percent of disorders, such as chronic fatigue syndrome and fibromyalgia are found in women. At first this seems quite strange, considering that, on average, females fight infection better than men and are known to naturally produce more antibodies. Possibly women differ in immune structure biologically due to child-bearing capacity and roles. In all likelihood, the evolution and development of societal functions also influence disease tendencies. Several decades ago, for example, the heart attack rate for women was much lower than for men. As gender roles changed, that gap has closed. Similarly, autoimmune disorders are not simply random accidents in the immune system; they do seem to be directed by some force and occur in a certain pattern.

I do not think that we can realistically attribute an autoimmune disorder to any one agent or cause; rather, it evolves from the interaction of many factors. The immune system has to exercise a certain amount of power in order to either reject altered cells or enhance healing: with the power to help also comes the power to harm. Is this one of the reasons I am seeing some of my strongest patients come down with some of the most severe chronic health issues? Disease can occur from unnecessary destruction of body tissue. And autoimmune diseases often arise from overly persistent healing. In other words, sometimes the immune system overdoes its job. In rheumatoid arthritis, joints are destroyed from unbridled healing, when pannus (scar tissue) invades the joints and bones. During kidney inflammation, the kidney's filters become clogged and damaged by unregulated or abnormal scar tissue in the skin, which forms scleroderma. In these types of cases, it seems as though the immune system gets "stuck in a rut" while carrying out a set of instructions; it does not know when to stop or to quit. Possibly there is a faulty form of communication or the pattern is off-kilter.

Often in people with autoimmune issues we also find repetitive thinking or mental chatter. This is also like getting stuck in a mental rut and spinning their wheels, but not going anywhere. We call this circular thinking. This stress appears to sometimes transform the immune system action into an autoimmune-style response.

We know that infection can play a decisive role in autoimmunity. Infections have been known to both trigger and prevent autoimmune reactions—at least in animal models. Take the example of specially bred mice in which up to 95 percent of the females develop diabetes, but if the mice have been previously exposed to infection, the number drops to 5–10 percent. It is as if the mice had a chance to practice an immune response with infection and then became more adept at controlling their own immune systems. But does the immune system work better with practice? Can we really compare a bodily system with a skill, such as learning to ride a bike? This seems unlikely; rather, it appears that the use of the immune system (and the communication systems involved) can be a learned response.

Could this model be applied to humans? Well that is a stretch, but we do know that in developed countries during the last fifty years, autoimmune-issue disorders have steadily increased.

Is the antiseptic environment of the modern family adding to the matrix of issues that lead to autoimmune problems? Are novel environmental and industrial toxins contributing to auto-immune disorders? Is our immune system and the ability to develop resistance to foreign substances (physical or emotional) like a muscle or the brain? In other words, does it need to be exercised in order to develop properly? Is the decreasing of child-hood disease coming back to haunt us in our adult life? There is no simple answer here, but these are all questions to be raised and factors to consider.

Most of these PNI and autoimmune issues are composed of psychological, neural and immunological attributes. As well, they all seem to involve a strong social aspect. How do these individuals perceive and cope with others in social situations? Are interactions in social settings the source of negative emotional experiences? The social action trigger appears to be as important, if not more, than the biological or psychological attributes in many autoimmune cases. For many, the onset of disease is closely linked to social and lifestyle factors, such as how busy they are, how much conflict is experienced in social interactions, the quality of their social support network and the degree to which they are able to process all this emotional experience.

In my practice I have seen a strong tendency toward perfec-tionism in those patients who have developed chronic fatigue syndrome (CFS) or fibromyalgia (FM). I have found several new studies, like one published by White (2000), *The Role of Person-ality in the Development and Perpetuation of Chronic Fatigue Syndrome*, which showed that CFS patients studied had a higher level of perfectionism than the control. It also reported that the CFS group reported a lower level of self-esteem than the control group. This sounded like what I was observing in my practice. The personality profiles of CFS and rheumatoid arthritis sufferers have also revealed similarities, and some researchers have even suggested that CFS resembles post-traumatic stress disorder. While we do not have a definitive personality profile at present, we can say there is a notable relationship between autoimmune health disorders such as CFS and FM and experiences of trauma, chronic stress and low self-esteem.

SUMMARY POINTS

1. Psychoneuroimmunology (PNI) shows that some health issues are partly psychological, neurological and immuno-logical. The center of gravity of a health issue can vary from person to person and from time to time within an individual.
2. There is direct communication between the nervous system and the immune system.
3. The immune system may act as a sense organ for the brain, influencing its function.
4. Day-to-day chronic stresses play a stronger role in immune function than one-time dramatic stress.
5. Contextual cues can trigger emotional memories that can produce immune responses.
6. Post-trauma syndrome (PTS) can highjack the nervous and immune systems.
7. The immune system can be conditioned or taught how to respond more effectively with practice.
8. We can create new coping skills to deal with and improve immune function.

9. Most people with genetic predispositions to disease will never develop the related issue. Even identical twins develop different coping skills for stress and, therefore, have different health outcomes.

10. Women develop far more autoimmune-related health issues than men.

11. In order to develop properly, the immune system needs to exercise.

12. There are several clear-cut social and psychological aspects to specific autoimmune disorders, such as chronic patterns of emotional stress, a driving personality style, difficulty coping with stress in social settings and low self-esteem.

Theory of Vibrational Medicine

CHAPTER FOUR

Energetic Dimensions of Vibrational Medicine

Jump-starting healing

Magnetic fields can "jump-start" the healing process in bone repair and move stalled healing energy even if the injury or disease dates back forty years. A fracture in the arm or leg that failed to heal within three to nine months would likely be treated with pulse electromagnetic field (PEMF) therapy. This small battery-powered pulse generator will induct a magnetic field around the bone, thus aiding the healing process.

We now find that electrical and magnetic field therapy is being successfully employed by the medical community for:

- Enhancement of capillary formation
- Decreased necrosis
- Reduced swelling
- Diminished pain
- Faster functional recovery
- Reduction in depth, area and pain in skin wounds
- Reduced muscle loss after ligament surgery
- Increased tensile strength of ligaments
- Acceleration of nerve regeneration and functional recovery

It has also been shown that early treatment with energy field therapy will enhance the body's ability to respond to an injury, while speeding up the healing process. What is it about the physical body that makes it so responsive to electromagnetic energy?

The living cellular matrix

In the traditional mechanical model of the body, cells were seen as a sacks of solutions, wherein the particles (enzymes, proteins, amino acids, sugars, etc.) were randomly diffused throughout the volume of the cell. When particular molecules happened to "bump into each other," their interactions created the chemical processes

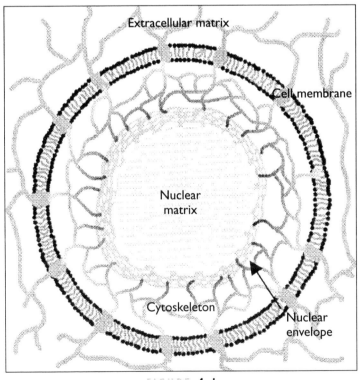

FIGURE 4.1

we called life. This "molecular soup" was considered definitive twenty years ago, with the assumption that the cell was nearly completely understood. Until recently, the discipline of biology fully subscribed to the soluble enzyme explanation of the cell.

We now know that the sack of solution explanation is not accurate. The cell is filled with filament, tubes, fibers and trabeculae—collectively called the cytoplasmic matrix or cytoskeleton—leaving little room for solutions of randomly diffusing "billiard ball" molecules. But more importantly, most of the water is bound in particular ways to the cellular framework, leaving very little water left for the so-called soluble enzyme idea of the molecular soup.

We now find that enzymes previously thought to be floating about within the cytoplasmic soup are actually attached to structures within the cell. To make this even more interesting, the cellular matrix is now believed to be connected across the cell surface. The connective tissue appears to create an extracelluar matrix (see Figure 4.1). Scientists have shown how the nuclear envelope, nuclear matrix and genes are continuously connected to all other cells through this cytoplasmic matrix. This means the boundary between the cell's exterior and the interior genetic material is not as sharply defined, nor as impermeable, as once thought. This continuous interconnected web extends throughout the entire body. So any therapeutic agent, be it physical touch, herbs, acupuncture, pharmaceuticals or electromagnetic frequency is able to contact the whole body. This matrix is called the connective tissue/cytoskeleton, the tissue-tensegrity matrix, or simply the living matrix.

Cells are not individual islands onto themselves. They are all interconnected. Groups of cells make up an organ system. Each organ system is analogous to a city: autonomous, but connected to other cities by many forms of communication and supply systems. The image of this large matrix of web-like interaction between every cell, tissue and organ puts a new perspective on the interaction of the therapist, therapeutic agent and the bodies to be worked on.

The type of communication in a living systems model of the physical body can be categorized into two main languages: chemical and energetic.

The chemical regulations are carried out by hormones and several secondary messengers within the cells. The energetic interactions can again be broken down into two types: electrical and electronic.

The electrical are large-scale actions like nerves and muscle activities; cells depolarize and then repolarize with ions such as sodium, potassium, chloride, calcium and magnesium. Electronic interactions are an area of new research. They deal with the flow of energy units much smaller than ions, such as electrons and electromagnetic waves.

As an analogy, we can compare the electrical actions in the body to the electricity that runs a home. The much smaller charges, in the form of semiconductors that control the electronics of a TV or computer, are like the electronic flow of communication in the body. In the computer, small amounts of power can perform extremely complex tasks. The electromagnetic waves are the information traveling from an entertainment system's remote control to the entertainment system or even the radio/TV waves coming into that system from the outside world. In humans and other living organisms, we are just beginning to investigate these forms of energy.

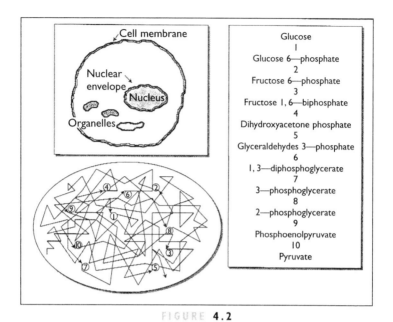

FIGURE **4.2**

Recently, there has been tremendous excitement about research into the world of the living cell matrix. A profound realization is occurring in the scientific community. The entire living matrix is perceived to be simultaneously a mechanical, vibrational or oscillatory, energetic, electronic and information network. Instead of thinking of the many cell reactions taking place in a solution, our understanding of the cell is more of a "solid state" biochemistry. The chemical reactions take place in the solid fibers and filaments that constitute a living cell (see Figure 4.2). This means that instead of the random pool ball theory of chemicals in a solution, we now consider cell interactions to be organized more like the pathways that speed the processes of electrons on a computer's electronic circuit board.

This also allows for the concept of communication signals that influence global control of the organism. We must consider not only the kind of chemical that is transferring energy but also the "vibration" or quality of the message being transferred.

For electronic communication to take place between a therapeutic agent and the body, the two need to be tuned into the same type of frequency. Just as one fine-tunes a radio to pick up the broadcast of a favorite station, it is believed that many herbal and homeopathic remedies are tuned into the human body "station" more closely than most pharmaceutical analogs. While synthetic substances (like most pharmaceuticals) work at the mechanical (biochemical) level, they are not able to resonate to a more subtle body frequency. However, substances such as herbal plant-based remedies, which have themselves developed through a "living" system, will be able to communicate both energetically as well as chemically.

Crystalline arrays in cells

When we think of crystals, we usually conceptualize them as hard solid material, like diamonds or quartz. Crystalline arrangements are very common in living systems and are found throughout the body. Living crystals are composed of long, thin, pliable molecules and are quite soft and flexible. In fact, living crystals are almost liquid, and when compressed and stretched, they generate electric fields. These very small electrical field generators convey information about the movement as well as contribute to the overall electromagnetic field surrounding the body (see Figure 4.3).

I remember my grandfather helping me build an old-fashioned crystal radio set when I was about seven years old. These sets were tuned to different stations or frequencies by moving the rod

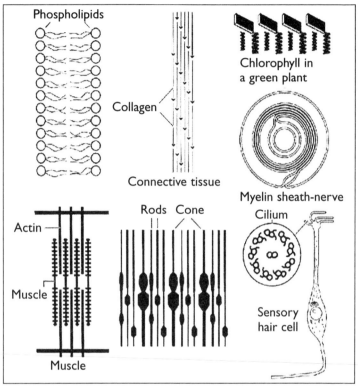

FIGURE 4.3

up and down on the crystal. The slightest movement of the body's living crystals can similarly tune into different frequencies and vibratory levels. This sensitivity is highly relevant for hands-on, energetic or movement therapies and the remedies that are used in vibrational medicine. Every stretch, massage or movement will change how a living crystal attunes to an aspect of the whole being. This is one of the reasons why tai chi, yoga, and hands-on therapies, such as Rolfing and Heller work, play a role in tuning

us into a clearer perception of our emotional and mental life—
and helps explain how acupuncture meridians and homeopathic
and botanical medicine work on an energetic nature. Because
these medicinal substances or modalities all have their own
living crystal structure, they too are sending out and receiving
specific frequencies. Once they have communicated within a
specific frequency range, all crystals tuned into that frequency
can receive the message. Therefore, if a botanical has a specific
frequency for the "liver" it can communicate with all parts along
the liver acupuncture meridian, because they are all tuned to the
same "radio station." This is what is meant when the old Chinese
masters say a herb enters the liver meridian.

Whacked in the head: seeing other bodies

In the early 1990s, I observed that the causes of problems for
many of my most sensitive patients went far beyond the physical.
Whether it was Chinook winds, solar flares and electromagnetic
disturbance or emotional stress, some of my patients were being
affected by these more subtle phenomena. I wondered what
proof we had for a vibrational theory of subtle body interactions.
I was certain that as humans we are composed of layers of subtle
bodies. I had experienced these subtle bodies and had direct
proof or knowledge of them proven to me by Grand Master Peng
in the late 1980s.

Grand Master Peng

After studying Chinese medicine and energetics for several
years, I became interested in Qi Chong (Chee Kong), an ancient
energy art that predates tai chi or kung fu. One of my associates
had contacts with a Grand Master of Qi Chong in Wuxi, China.

Qi Chong is an ancient art of energy (qi) flow and was either used for healing or as a martial art. Peng was given the title of Grand Master because he was the trainer of masters in Qi Chong. He was credited with many "miraculous" healing feats. I was curious and decided to see him firsthand, but one thing led to another and I was unable to take time away from the clinic or the college, so I delayed my trip. My colleagues suggested we put energy into bringing him to Canada instead of me going to China. We did, and after six months of red tape, I finally met Grand Master Peng.

Different masters, I learned, had different "talents." Grand Master Peng practiced a form of soft Qi Chong, used for healing people. Besides this, his talent was subtle vision. He could see energy fields very well.

My goal was to study both Grand Master Peng and to study with him for six to twelve months, the length of his visa. So, every morning a small group of us got up at 6:00 am and went through a series of classes—all conducted through a translator, as Peng spoke no English and we no Chinese. The classes included both theory and exercises from the Shaolin Temple tradition. As far as Peng seeing patients, I sent him a steady stream, but did not advertise him, as his techniques were unusual for Calgary in the 1980s. His method was to simply gaze at a patient, assess his or her problems and explain that he was tuning into different frequencies. The Master could see either clouds of mismatched energy or acupuncture points that were the wrong color. This told him the nature of the illness and its location in the body. Usually the patient would lie down on a massage table and he would look at them while he passed his hands about six inches over the body. Then he would move his hands in particular patterns and direct energy toward the patient. It seemed pretty safe and almost too simple. But before long we realized that he could not use the clinic's treatment rooms: because his energy was too strong he often had to move twelve to twenty feet back from the patient when he directed the healing energy—the only way he could lessen the energy before it entered the patient. For months, a steady stream of patients with every kind of complaint came to visit Master Peng.

During these first few weeks I gained confidence in Peng's abilities, so I sent him more difficult cases, including one women who had a visibly hardened lump of breast cancer. For her own personal reasons she had refused surgery and chemotherapy, and had decided to work on it naturally. Within a week of treatments, the lump seemed to disappear. How could that be? Grand Master Peng was pushing the envelope of my healing models, but I was intrigued. During this whole time "Project Qi Chong" was kept quiet, as we had the reputation of both the clinic and the college to preserve. But this patient had a girlfriend in Edmonton who also had breast cancer. She was the wife of a very prominent political figure. After seeing Master Peng, her body was rid of breast cancer. Enthusiastically, she was determined to spread the word and go public. So, within one month of the start of Grand Master Peng's secret study group, he found himself interviewed (with a translator) on CBC TV news, and in two local newspapers. Within another week, he had a waiting list of more than 900 people with every kind of health problem, all hoping to be healed.

During the following month, I was traveling on the lecture circuit and on my return noticed an energy drain in Peng. The receptionists were sending people in on a critical-need basis, and I recognized how this was draining him. We immediately

PART TWO ☆ Theory of Vibrational Medicine

changed that, so instead of sending fifteen critically ill patients to him every day, we selected a mix of patients with problems like arthritis and high blood pressure, rather than filling the entire day with life-threatening problems. That seemed to help, but I decided to take him up to Banff's hot springs the next weekend for some relaxation. I figured a few hours in an outdoor hot mineral pool on a wintry day would help rejuvenate anyone, so off we went.

It was one of those magical days when the steam off the pool interacted with the cold air and light, falling snow to create a gentle mist that hung over the pool. Peng, his translator, and another student and I had been soaking our muscles for more than an hour in the pool. I was enjoying myself and Peng had a big smile on his face. I turned to adjust my position against the edge of the pool and wham, Peng slapped me hard on the back of the head. Confused, I reached for something to hang onto and almost slid under the water. Why had he hit me? Both Peng and his translator continued soaking. I glanced his way, but he made no attempt to explain himself. The pool became still and soon a sense of contentment settled over us. I looked out at the mountain backdrop and the world took on a pink glow in the mist. Still a little shaken by the hit on the head, we got out and under Peng's guidance did some of our exercises in the changing room. The spectacle disturbed other patrons so, we finished dressing and left in silence. I pointed the car toward the Banff Springs Hotel, which looked like a beautiful medieval castle against the white mountain peaks. With no discussion, the translator pulled us into a medium-sized, deserted conference room and we continued with our exercises. As we performed the set of movements, Peng came up to each of us and, with his knuckles closed in a drilling action, squeezed pressure into the palms of our hands and our foreheads, or "third eye." After he had finished this, he stood behind each of us and whacked us all on the head. I saw him whack the other two first, so this time I was ready. Although it was part of his teaching techniques, a whack on the head still hurt.

When our exercises finished, we walked out of the room into the mezzanine area where we could look down onto the lobby. Grabbing the railing, I squinted and tried to adjust my eyes. For a minute I felt light-headed and was no longer seeing people. All I could see were these large Jell-O-like egg shapes, bobbing along in the lobby. I had spent enough time studying esoteric literature to know what I was witnessing. I was seeing peoples' subtle bodies. Like transparent Russian dolls, I could see through the outer layer into the next layer and the next layer, each one a little denser than the one extending beyond it. Counting the layers, I believe I saw four egg-like envelopes around each person crossing the lobby. I looked at Peng and grinned. He had been so happy with his hot springs adventure that he wanted to show us how he saw the world. During the next few days, one body at a time started to disappear, until by the fourth day, I could no longer see the energy bodies. Peng's gift was gone and my sight returned to normal. What an experience and yes, ever since then, I have tried to convince him to hit me again, but that was the one and only time.

This experience proved to me that the other energy bodies do exist. Wanting to know more about their composition and how I could use this information to help work with my patients, I went back to my notes on vibrational medicine and began to review the theories of William Tiller, Richard Gerber, Michael Talbot and Einstein.

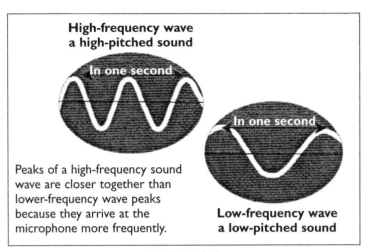

FIGURE **4.4**

The dimensions of vibrational medicine

Physicists explain that the material world we live in is really a huge electromagnetic soup. Two simple examples of vibrational energy within the electromagnetic spectrum are sound waves that resonate at a frequency that stimulates our ears to hear, and light waves that reveal the words on this page. However, there are many other vibrational wavelengths that we have to manipulate to perceive. The electromagnetic spectrum is represented by waves of varying frequencies (see Figure 4.4). The highest frequencies are X-rays and gamma rays. Microwaves, radio waves, heat and visible light represent lower frequencies. At the lowest end of the spectrum is electrical power—60 cycles per second, known as power-frequency. As can be seen in Figure 4.5 there is a broad spectrum of various wavelengths. All of these frequencies take up what appears to be the same space. Electromagnetic fields carry energy through space.

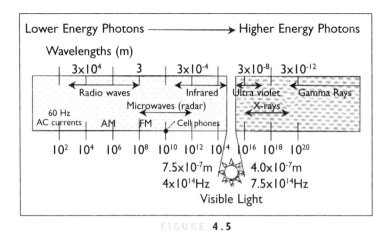

FIGURE 4.5

The same antenna can pick up not only AM/FM radio and television, but can be tuned to many different channels, each of which registers different wavelengths. All these wavelengths still take up the same "space/time."

Vibrational medicine is both the awareness and the application of vibrational energies to improve and maintain health. The application takes into consideration all the many forms and frequencies of vibrational energy that contribute to the multi-dimensional experience we call life. Einstein's famous formula ($E=mc^2$) proved that matter and energy are not only actually interconvertible and interchangeable, they are two different expressions of the same thing. This statement has stood the test of time and the rigors of contemporary research.

Matter is like a frozen form of energy. Just as ice vibrates at a slower frequency than water, and much slower than steam, our physical reality is a combination of frozen energy vibrations, all moving at different speeds/frequencies. The human energy field is partially made up of atoms and subatomic particles that are a form of frozen energy, or matter, vibrating more slowly than other subtle forms of energy. This might sound a bit esoteric at first, but it is part of an evolving knowledge of how our bodies work. Hospitals currently use aspects of "vibrational medicine" in the form of diagnostic tools that use technology to measure these frequencies, such as electrocardiograms (EKGs) that record the "energy patterns" of the heart; magnetic resonance imaging (MRI), used to obtain microscopic chemical and physical data; X-rays and ultrasounds.

The concept of the body as a complex energetic system is slowly gaining scientific acceptance. While acupuncture and qi energy or Ayurveda have been widely used in other cultures for millennia, the West has been slow to embrace these energetic medical models. There is a gradual integration of these models into some medical practitioners' model and even into some hospitals' repertoires.

The newly emerging model of vibrational or energy medicine in no way refutes the validity of biomechanical and biological knowledge of the physical body; rather, it builds on that material to create a model that works with a broader picture of the electromagnetic fields we live in. The physical body's cells are fed by a continuous stream of nutrients and chemical responses and by an electromagnetic force or life-force energy. In other cultures, this life force energy goes by many names, such as qi, (chi, chee), ki, prana and vital energy. While knowledge of these systems is not new, a framework for using them together with modern medicine is.

Many energetic medical models have shown that there are specific pathways for energy distribution, such as acupuncture meridians and chakra systems, that support the cells and organs of the body. These systems can enhance or inhibit the flow of life energy, and shifts in that flow are affected by a multitude of factors: emotional, mental and/or physical. Finding a means to include these systems in our evolving model of health is essential. Emotions, the quality of our relationships and even faith in a universal being can affect the flow of this energy.

Vibrational medicine shows that consciousness itself is not just a by-product of physical and biochemical mechanisms, but plays a primary role in health and illness. While biomechanical medicine has been looking for that part of the brain that controls consciousness and thought, vibrational medicine accepts that such awareness takes place in an entirely different energy field. You wouldn't take apart a radio to try and find Beethoven when you hear his *Fifth Symphony*. Well, vibrational medicine looks at the brain like a radio receiver that receives information from the emotional and mental body. In other words, we are not simply sophisticated meat machines, with biocomputer brains and nervous systems; we are conscious beings with physical bodies that are only one dimension of our existence.

A vital component of the vibrational medicine model is that of communication. We now know the cells also communicate with each other by a nonchemical means. How this is accomplished is still being researched, but in all probability it is by some electromagnetic means. Cells actually emit weak pulses of light that seem to form the basis of an indeterminate communication system. Apparently, there is some inherent mechanism in a cell that decodes information presented by other cells, which means there is a communication system that exists outside the realms of chemistry and receptor sites. All of the answers for how the body, or even more specifically we as complex beings, communicate, cannot be answered by chemistry alone. There are other fields of communication. For example, how do fish swim together or birds fly in tight formation without bumping into each other? There seems to be some inherent form of communication system operating.

We see this kind of "pacemaker" activity in various parts of our physical body. Most of us are familiar with the concept of a pacemaker in the heart, but the cells of the digestive tract and the urinary tract also have coordinating fields that keep the movements in harmony with each other. They all seem to be marching to the beat of the same drummer. This drummer is the life energy or vital energy that leaves the body when we die.

From a mechanical point of view, when we die, all is over. The physical body decays and is recycled into other organisms in the biosphere. The personality and all that we are stops existing. In the vibrational medicine model, the belief is that the life force moves on after death, storing the experiences it had in this lifetime. The spirit directs or animates the physical body to aid us in relating to others, to gain knowledge and create in the physical plane, but the spirit exists in dimensions beyond this plane. We can say this is similar to the way a driver directs an automobile.

We believe that many other dimensions exist, and are explored in sleep and dream states. We are really spiritual beings with our roots in this physical world in order to experience its lessons. We are multidimensional beings having a physical experience.

Currently, many practitioners find that by working with a larger energy vibrational model, which includes spiritual concepts, they can more easily find ways to assist the healing process. With the proper training and lots of patience, most can learn how to perceive these subtle energies. Two of the most recognized and accepted energy systems are acupuncture and chakra.

Acupuncture — meridian system

The art and science of acupuncture dates back thousands of years, with some of the first written records being 5,000 years old. In China, by 3000 BC, it was already a well established discipline. The modern form of acupuncture is starting to gain both acceptance and use in Western society. Many progressive medical doctors are referring patients to acupuncturists, and some are incorporating acupuncture into their practice. Acupuncture is based on the concept of life energy called qi. Throughout the body, qi flows in channels or meridians, which distribute this life energy to all the cells. The acupuncturist's role is to assist the qi's proper flow and regulate it by inserting fine needles into specific points. These acupuncture points are unique areas, located just below the skin on the meridians, that have been shown to influence the flow of qi and thus affect the whole body down to the cellular level. Disease, in terms of traditional Chinese medicine, is an imbalance of the qi to the various organs of the body. By rebalancing the qi, the acupuncturist brings the body back into a state of better health. Acupuncturists also use diet, herbs, exercise, moxibustion (burning a herb over an acupuncture point), cupping and counseling.

In traditional Chinese medicine, an individual's health comprises of two basic forms of qi: prenatal and postnatal.

Prenatal qi is the energy with which individuals are born, and is inherited from the parents.

Postnatal qi can be divided thus:

Qi obtained from diet and medicines—nutrient qi

Qi that results from interaction with the environment—environmental qi.

The latter can either be spent or accumulated depending on the type of interaction. This makes the acupuncture points a two-way communication system, or portal, between an individual and the electromagnetic soup we live in.

Chakra system

The word "chakra" comes from Sanskrit, meaning "wheel." There are several types of chakra systems imported from the East; the primary ones are from India and Tibet. The simplest and most commonly used in the West is based on seven chakras, which are considered portal systems, similar to the acupuncture points, but of higher intensity. They transfer or communicate life energies between the various bodies. Vortexes of vibrational energy, the chakras swirl around in a wheel-like fashion, transmitting what Hindus call prana: a vibrational energy occurring on a different vibrational level than qi, and affected mostly by our emotional and spiritual development. The energy or "vibrational information" that travels through these chakra vortexes is emotional and what the yogis call spiritual. The chakra system is now being studied by many in the West and is employed in healing models by numerous practitioners.

Each of the chakras is associated with a specific gland, nerve bundle or ganglion (collection of nerve cells) of the endocrine system. In a way, these areas are like mini-brains. Each chakra processes specific types of emotional, relationship and spiritual information. The bodily location of the chakra also seems to hold emotional memory. This often means that we remember emotional detail as much, if not more, with our body as our mind-brain. Healthy, emotional flow will stimulate and feed the chakras, while emotional stagnation and anomalies will congest the flow of energy. Thus, stress-related symptoms that appear in the physical body are often the manifestation of "energy problems" that occur as disturbances at a higher, or more subtle, energy level.

There are some researchers who can see disturbances in our energy fields. One very popular author, Carolyn Myss, is reported to have a 93 percent accuracy rate for detecting the emotional and mental precursors to disease in the energy field around a person. She feels that the majority of disease and illness results from overload of unresolved emotional, psychological and spiritual crises. Myss describes these energy fields using the chakra system based on seven major chakra centers with several minor chakras. The following is an explanation of the major centers and the physical and emotional issues associated with these vortex centers.

First or root chakra, located at the base of the spine, is associated with survival, safety and security and our connectedness to the earth or being grounded. This area is connected in a minor way to the reproductive system, but more to the hip joints, lower back and pelvic area. This includes lower back pain, sciatica, legs, varicose veins, bones, rectal difficulties, some forms of depression and some cancers (e.g., prostate), as well as certain immune functions. Mental and emotional issues that arise from the first chakra include family and group safety, the ability to provide for life's necessities, ability to stand up for self, feeling at home, and social and familial law and order. Paranoia, belongingness or feelings of being threatened can influence this area.

Second or sacral chakra resides in the pelvic area and has a strong connection to the sexual organs, emotional expression, and personal power—in terms of business and social relationships. The emotional feelings associated with this energy frequency usually involve sexuality and self-worth, some forms of creative expression, and a sense of ethics and honor in relationships. When a person perceives self-worth as external measures of money, job and sexuality only, we often find a distortion in this area. Obsession with material gain is often considered the other side of the low self-worth coin. Malfunction in this area can affect the reproductive system. Problems that might manifest are menstrual difficulties, infertility, vaginal infections, ovarian cysts, impotency, lower back pain, hip pain, large intestine disorders, appendicitis, pelvic and sexual dysfunction, slipped disks and bladder and urinary infections. It should be noted that even though dysfunction in this or any chakra can cause these problems, the opposite is not necessarily true. If a person has a bladder infection, it does not guarantee there is a problem with his or her second chakra. There are many other circumstances that may cause a bladder infection.

Third or solar plexus chakra energetically feeds the digestive tract, including the abdomen, small intestine, gall-bladder, kidneys, liver, pancreas, adrenal glands and spleen. This energy level, not to be confused with self-worth, has to do with self-confidence, self-respect and empowerment. The concept of "gut feeling" and personal power often has to do with the energy of this chakra. The instinct, "this doesn't feel right" comes from this level. Blockage of energy in the solar plexus chakra can cause ulcers, cancerous tumors, diabetes, hepatitis, anorexia, bulimia and other stomach-related problems. Author Caroline Myss suggests that the enculturation of fear and issues of unresolved anger are believed to be deeply connected to physical dysfunction in this body region. Trust, care for oneself and others, responsibility for making decisions, sensitivity to criticism and personal honor all relate to this chakra.

Fourth or heart chakra resides in the middle of the chest and is associated with the thymus, the immune system and the heart; it is considered one of the most important energy centers of the body, representing the ability to express love as well as nurture, and the ability to feel affinity with other beings. Its energies charge the organic heart. Feelings of unresolved anger and expression of conditional love will impact the healthy functioning of the heart.

The original cause of heart problems may or may not be caused by congestion of the fourth chakra. However, work on the heart chakra has been shown to improve the recovery rate of heart attack patients and those who have atherosclerotic plaque in the heart and vessels. Cardiologist, Dr. Dean Ornish, used a combination of exercise, diet and a type of meditation called "open heart meditation" to open the heart chakra. There was a complete reversal of atherosclerotic plaque in the subjects studied.

Besides the heart, the fourth chakra also influences the lungs, breast, diaphragm, ribs, shoulders and arms. Symptoms of a blocked heart chakra include heart attacks, enlarged heart, asthma, allergies, lung cancer, bronchial issues, circulation problems and problems associated with upper back and shoulders. The thymus, and thus the T-lymphocytes of the immune system, is closely linked to the heart chakra.

Fifth or throat chakra is associated with the thyroid, parathyroid, mouth, vocal cord, trachea, neck vertebra and esophagus, and represents personal expression as a reflection of communication, creativity, purpose of life and willpower. Problems represented in this area include chronic throat problems, muscular and nerve problems of the jaw (TMJ), throat and mouth cancer, stiffness of the neck, thyroid dysfunction and migraines. Caroline Myss points out that creativity and self-expression are essential for one's health. She adds that an inability to express one's feelings, whether it be joy, sorrow, anger or love, is similar to pouring concrete down your throat, thus closing off the energy needed to sustain the health of the region.

Sixth or brow or third-eye chakra is situated in the forehead, above and between the eyes and is associated with intuition, discrimination, the ability to access wisdom, self-evaluation, truth, feeling of adequacy, openness to the ideas of others, ability to learn from experience and emotional intelligence. Connected to the pituitary and pineal gland, eyes, ears, nose and the nervous system, it charges the intellect and reasoning skills. Intuition from the sixth chakra is more of a universal quality rather than the personal gut level experience of the solar plexus chakra. Problems in this area are associated with brain tumors, hemorrhages, strokes, blindness, neurological disturbance, comas, depression, schizophrenia, deafness, learning disabilities and seizures.

Seventh or crown chakra is the energy represented by the halo in Christian religions. When this area is fully functioning the person is open to his or her "higher self." The area is also related to the muscular and skeletal systems, as well as the skin. Problems in this field have to do with energetic disorders, mystical depression, chronic exhaustion that has no physical link and extreme sensitivities to light, sound and other environmental factors. The mental and emotional issues that rise from this chakra are the ability to trust life; knowing one's values, ethics and courage; humanitarianism; selflessness; ability to see large patterns; faith and inspiration; and spirituality and devotion.

Different experiences in our psychospiritual life (both positive and negative) will influence the various areas of our body associated with those frequencies. For instance, if we have difficulty dealing with personal power, this will influence the flow of energy through the associated vortex constricting energy flow to the third chakra area. Even though the area of chakra influence is not recognized by modern medicine, it greatly influences our health and overall energy level. This does not mean that diet, herbs, exercise and other factors do not play an important role in the health issue, just that the chakra influence should be equally considered when determining the cause of a disorder.

The research being done by mainstream medicine into energy medicine is steadily gaining ground. One notable contributor is Valerie Hunt from the University of California, who started measuring the electromagnetic frequency of muscle, but shifted to a study of the chakra frequencies. She was fascinated that the frequency of the chakra centers (1600 cycles per second [cps]) was much higher than could be explained by even the heart and the brain frequencies (0–250 cps). Finding these energy vortexes—that represented much higher frequencies than those found anywhere else in the body—motivated her to further research the chakra system.

When considering the chakras, envision them as hose faucets or, more accurately, lenses that let energy through. When the lens is more open, more electromagnetic or magneoelectric energy flows in. Chakras are always active, providing energy from more subtle bodies that represent emotional and mental energies that

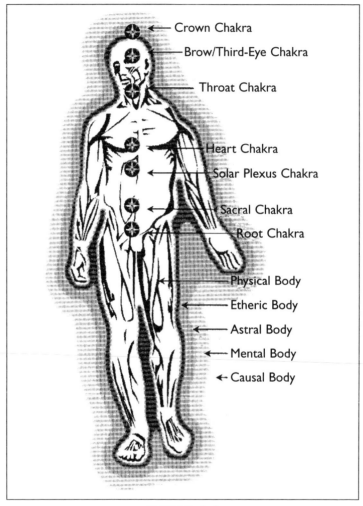

FIGURE **4.6**

we will discuss later. However, if there is constriction in this lens, not much energy is able to flow to that particular physical area, and the person cannot integrate the emotional/social attributes of that chakra. Thus, health issues arise. If the chakra is too open and the person cannot integrate that energy pattern, problems can also develop.

Because the chakras provide the connection for the emotions to the physical level, emotional problems can create an imbalanced flow in the energy transfer system. By becoming knowledgeable in the language of the chakra system, individuals can use this unique emotional and spiritual feedback to aid in determining influences in a health issue. As well as developing a fuller model for the multidimensional human being, we will be able to see how these energies affect our daily lives.

We wear many bodies

Besides the physical body and the energy systems that contribute to health, we have several other bodies. These bodies are (see Figure 4.6):

- Etheric
- Astral
- Mental
- Causal

This system of bodies has been taught in the East for millennia, and conscious contact with these higher frequencies is likely what the Christian mystical tradition referred to as "transverberation."

The etheric body is surrounding and interpenetrating our physical body. Because it is of a higher vibrational rate, it can take up what appears to be the same "space" as the physical body. It is invisible to the normal human eye, but can be seen by clairvoyants and photographed using Kirlian photography. The etheric body is a basic blueprint or, as some consider it, a mold for our physical body. This template aids in directing the structure, spacing and function of the physical body. Some think of the etheric body as a Jell-O mold that guides cell growth into the right location.

Since the etheric body is a template, any disturbance of its electromagnetic field can be translated into anomalies in the physical body. This concept fits well with traditional Chinese medicine that teaches imbalances in the qi flow will sooner or later affect the physical body. Many feel that the etheric body directly influences the acupuncture meridians and that it is the location of these pathways. The chakra system uses the etheric body as the interface with the physical for the more subtle bodies.

The astral body is influenced by emotions. Some call it the emotional body, and it is the expression of how we feel and express ourselves. The astral body is on an even higher vibrational magnetic frequency than the etheric body. More mobile than the etheric body, the astral body is strongly attracted to the physical body. Astral projection is the movement of the astral body and is experienced by many at night when they have "traveling" or "flying" dreams. The extent to which the chakras' lenses are open will determine the amount and clarity of emotional information transferred. Disturbances in the emotional body easily influence the energy systems of the physical body.

The mental body is a field of subtle magnetic energy, vibrating faster than the astral body. Thought (conscious or unconscious), creativity, inventions and inspiration originate from this level. Disturbances in the mental body can cause energy anomalies that will eventually filter down into the physical body, usually via and colored by the emotional world.

The causal body or causal field is often considered the soul: the area where everything experienced on the physical plane, both in this lifetime and others, is recorded. It is also considered the location of the "higher self," the wiser part of people that sees things in the light of a universal picture. The causal body reflects reincarnations and the archetypal knowledge of the journey taken on a spiritual sojourn to obtain experiences on the physical plane. Disturbances from this level can be as simple as a birthmark or involve dramatic health, emotional and social issues.

The production of emotional disturbance found in the astral body is the accumulation of "emotional baggage" that goes unresolved in the emotional realm. Vibrational medicine shows that these anomalies on the emotional level can be translated down to the physical level and decoded at the molecular level to cause biochemical changes in the body. Gerber states in his fascinating book *Vibrational Medicine*: "Thoughts are particles of energy. Thoughts are accompanied by emotions which also begin at the energy levels. As these particles of energy filter through from the etheric level to the physical level, the end result is immuno-incompetence." We often find that it is emotional processing that breaks down first or creates a split in our body's communication system.

Communication between the physical and the astral body is via the chakra system using the etheric interface as its portal system. It is via this interface of the etheric body that the chakras supply information to the physical realm from the astral body.

SUMMARY POINTS

1. All parts of our body are connected in a continuously flowing communication system. Blocks in that communication system can cause disease.

2. Communication can be chemical or energetic. The energetic communication can be further broken down into electrical and electronic.
3. The whole living matrix can be perceived as simultaneously a mechanical, vibrational, oscillatory, energetic and electronic information network.
4. Living crystals, which form many parts of our connective tissue, generate electric fields that convey information about the pattern of movement. They contribute to the overall electromagnetic field surrounding our body.
5. Many therapeutic modalities work as much on an energetic level as they do on a physical chemical level.
6. Qi Chong is a form of vibrational energy healing that is very effective for many people.
7. Physics shows us that the entire universe is made up of various electromagnetic frequencies. Because these frequencies vibrate at different wavelengths, they can take up the same space.
8. Einstein proved that physical matter is really frozen energy with its own vibrational frequency.
9. The universe is composed of far more than only mechanical parts. It is filled with vital energy that also flows through us.
10. We are spiritual beings having a physical experience.
11. The acupuncture meridians are one of the energy communication systems of the vital energy or qi that circulates in the body.
12. We have at least seven chakras that work as energy stations, representing various emotional or psychological

states. Imbalance in these areas can contribute to health issues in associated parts of the body.

13. We have a physical body, along with etheric, emotional (astral), mental and spiritual bodies.

14. To find out what created a health issue, we have to determine its center of gravity. We must establish both which body the issue resides in (physical, astral, mental) and the influence of the various energy communication systems, such as chakra or acupuncture meridians.

CHAPTER FIVE

Tiller Model of Subtle Bodies and Holograms

❖

The Tiller Model

In 1988, when Richard Gerber, MD, first published his book *Vibrational Medicine: New Choices for Healing Ourselves,* I discovered the ideas of William Tiller, Ph.D., Professor Emeritus and Head of the department of Material Science and Engineering, Stanford University.

Tiller created a mathematical model of the various subtle bodies and how they relate to both this three-dimensional world and other dimensions. While I was not completely unfamiliar with this model—since it had been circulating among the homeopathic community for some time—Tiller explained its complexity in the clearest way. Holistic health practitioners, especially those practicing homeopathy, found these ideas (that there is a tangible relationship between this and other dimensions) helped explain how a medicine, which was so diluted as to be undetectable, still yielded results in their patients. The model is fascinating and highly detailed; here I will give just a brief overview. You can get a more detailed look at it in Gerber's *Vibrational Medicine: New Choices for Healing Ourselves* or from Tiller's books: *Science and Human Transformation: Subtle Energies, Intentionality and Consciousness* and *Conscious Acts of Creation: The Emergence of a New Physics.*

Tiller starts with a simple model of how most doctors, including allopathic physicians, look at a person:

Function ⟷ Structure ⟷ Chemistry

The equation shows that all functions of the body arise from the structure (anatomy) of the body, as determined by the chemistry of the situation. This means that there is always a chemical reason for anything that is generated by or that affects our bodies. In other words, whenever there is a malfunction, there is a chemical imbalance that creates the structural and functional defect. This view of health collapses the physical, emotional or mental issues into one level of functioning.

More recently, there has been an increasing awareness of the influence of electromagnetic fields, so the equation has been expanded to:

Function ⟷ Structure ⟷ Chemistry ⟷ Electro-magnetic Energy Fields

---

Small electromagnetic fields have been shown to aid in the healing of bones and other parts of the body. However, the equation still falls short—in showing how holistic practitioners would perceive healing—because it ignores the energies of the subtle energy fields, and the influence of immeasurable things like homeopathy and flower essences.

Tiller developed a more sophisticated equation that takes into account the field of vibrational medicine.

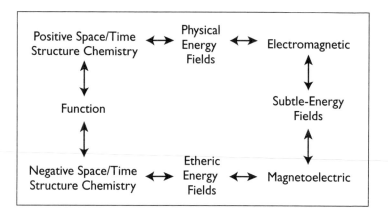

At first this equation might appear rather strange. Allopathy uses the upper part of the equation and homeopathy the lower. This equation proposes to unite the two disciplines with this schemata of energy communication. The electromagnetic fields interact with the more subtle bodies (etheric, astral and mental) that seem to be in the magnetoelectric energy field range (this will be explained later). These fields also interact with our etheric chemistry, which functions in negative space/time (−S/T) or as an invisible structure that interacts with physical function. To quote Tiller:

> We are all elements of spirit, indestructible and eternal, and multi-dimensional in the divine. We contain a unique mechanism of perfection which is mind....
>
> This mind creates a vehicle for experience (a universe, a word, a body) and each person, as a spiritual being plus perception mechanism, invests in that vehicle which runs a continuously programmed course. The being is connected to the vehicle via the emotional circuitry. The stuff used for construction of this vehicle or *simulator* is of dual or conjugate nature. One part, which is electrical in nature and travels at velocities less than that of electromagnetic light, is of positive energy and positive mass. It forms the *physical* part of the simulator. The other part, which is magnetic in nature and travels at velocities greater than that of electromagnetic light, is a negative mass, and negative energy. It forms the *etheric* parts of the simulator. The total sum of these two energies is zero, as is the sum of their entropies. Thus, the total simulator or vehicle is created out of what we call 'empty space,' the space of mind, via fluctuation type of process."

Tiller-Einstein and Gerber

To understand this whole concept, we have to go further into the Tiller-Einstein model, as Gerber calls it. We will turn to the Gerber overview for insight. The explanation comes from the famous equation, $E=mc^2$. A more accurate version of the equation is modified by a proportionality constant known as the Einstein-Lorentz Transformation. This makes the formula look more like (see Figure 5.1):

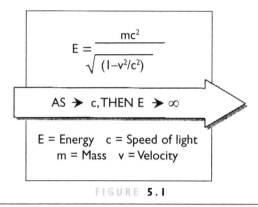

$$E = \frac{mc^2}{\sqrt{(1-v^2/c^2)}}$$

AS ➤ c, THEN E ➤ ∞

E = Energy   c = Speed of light
m = Mass   v = Velocity

FIGURE **5.1**

The classical interpretation of this is that the energy contained in a particle is equivalent to its mass (weight), times the speed of light squared. This shows us that even a very small particle contains an awesome amount of energy (as observed with the atomic bomb). As we said earlier, it also shows that energy and mass are interchangeable and that physical reality is just "frozen" energy. If one speeds up a particle faster and faster, until it approaches the speed of light, its kinetic energy increases exponentially as described by the equation: Kinetic Energy $= mv^2$ where "v" is velocity. You can see this in Figure 5.2.

This equation is one of the reasons that most physicists believe that it is impossible to go faster than the speed of light because, to go faster than the speed of light, you would have to find the square root of a negative number (e.g., −1). Mathematicians call these imaginary numbers and most physicists do not believe in the imaginary number set, as abstract mathematicians do. However, mathematicians like Charles Muses believe that the square root of negative numbers produce what he calls "hypernumbers," which

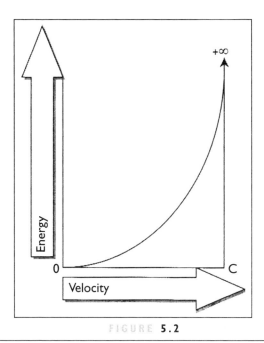

FIGURE **5.2**

he believes describe the behavior of higher dimensional phenomena (such as subtle bodies). If we put biases aside for a moment and follow Muses' train of thought, we get an interesting graph, which is a mirror image of the first graph (see Figure 5.3).

Negative entropy

The top left-hand part of the graph is what Tiller calls the positive space/time (+S/T) structure that we see on a day-to-day basis. This is the material that exists at speeds slower than the speed of light. The inverted curve in the lower right-hand side is Tiller's negative space/time (–S/T). These particles move faster than the speed of light, taking up no space. Because these particles travel

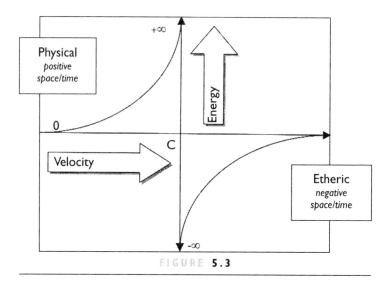

FIGURE **5.3**

faster than the speed of light, we can't see them, as we see only what reflects light back to our eyes. Some physicists have theorized about this group of particles and call them tachyons. The properties of the supraluminal (faster than light) would not fit in the electromagnetic spectrum (EM). Particles that are negative space/time matter would be, in Tiller's terms, "magnetoelectric" (ME). What is even more significant than this faster-than-light material is that since it takes up negative mass, that would mean that it has negative entropy. This becomes very significant, as entropy is a term that is used to describe the tendency toward disorder. Almost everything in the physical universe tends toward positive entropy and falls apart.

Things in the physical world are in a constant process of decay. There is one major exception to that rule and that is living systems. While everything is decaying, biological systems take in raw material (food) and organize it into more complex components. As Gerber writes, "Living systems display the property of negative entropy or a tendency toward decreasing disorder of the system." The energy that seems to animate our physical being is in a process of negative entropy.

Does this equation describe the concept of vital energy, or qi, that is described in natural healing from many cultures and medical models throughout history? Qi is characterized by negative entropy and belongs to the etheric negative space/time quadrant of Tiller's model. As soon as we take away this vital energy, we snuff out the vital force, and the physical body enters positive entropy and decays like the rest of the physical components of the physical universe. We are suggesting the etheric body $(-S/T)$ directs the flow of energy to animate the physical body $(+S/T)$.

This opens up all kinds of possibilities. The etheric body is beyond the speed of light, so that we cannot see it unless we are sensitive to these frequencies. Since the astral body is more subtle than the etheric body, it exists at an even faster vibration. Both move at speeds above that of electromagnetic light. Tiller considers that the astral body operates at speeds between 10^{10} and 10^{20} times the speed of light.

Just as we have physical parts to our physical body, we have emotional forms in the astral body. Clairvoyants have described these unique hues and shapes as color fields. This means that there can be energy flows and blocks of that flow in our astral body similar to blockages in the physical body. Because of the magnetic energy of the astral (faster-than-light) body, it would tend to be more mercurial, pulsating and moving in more than one direction at a time, like the Jell-O-shaped eggs around bodies that I saw in my few short days of etheric sight. It appears that this magnetic energy tends to attract others who are in harmony with it and repel those who are not. The old saying "misery loves company" comes to mind. Is this how we are attracted to a certain crowd? This also shows us another look at Sheldrake's morphic resonance idea. Does attraction happen at a magnetic level and involve the other subtle bodies?

This, of course, means that many therapeutic agents like herbals, homeopathics and flower essences could deliver some or all of their therapeutic energies via the magnetoelectric circuitry, instead of via purely chemical means, as with pharmaceuticals. All of this suggests that the realms of physics and mathematics might already have within their grasp a way to define the subtle bodies through the positive-negative space/time model, based on Einstein's original theory of relativity.

The body that resides above or beyond the astral (emotional) body is the mental body, which resides at an even higher frequency. For the mental (or intellect) body to communicate with the phys-ical body, it first sends the information to, or through, the astral body, then the etheric body, and finally to the physical body. In this process, the mental concepts literally filter through the emotions; therefore, most, if not all, of our mental concepts are colored by our emotions. Of course, mental concepts that are in this subtle mental body have to be "stepped down" to be perceived by our brain and other circuitry of the physical body—which means that we are not always getting a clear image of what the mental body is "thinking" or processing. Such an image would be a bit fuzzy.

Figure 5.4 shows Tiller's model in simplistic graphic form. It is not that different than the model of the bodies discussed in the previous chapter except for the mental body. In the Tiller model we see three separate mental bodies.

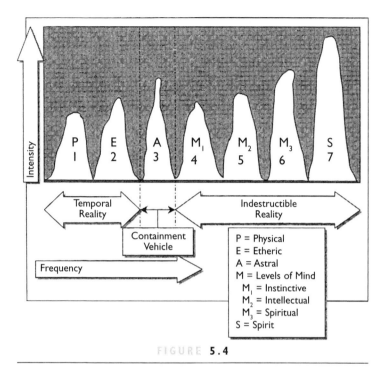

P
I
E
2
A
3
M₁
4
M₂
5
M₃
6
S
7

Intensity

Temporal Reality

Indestructible Reality

Containment Vehicle

Frequency

P = Physical
E = Etheric
A = Astral
M = Levels of Mind
  M₁ = Instinctive
  M₂ = Intellectual
  M₃ = Spiritual
S = Spirit

FIGURE **5.4**

M_1—representing instinctive functions

M_2—representing intellectual functions

M_3—representing lower spiritual functions

Outside this level of mind we have the dimension of causal body (spiritual) that some call the "higher self." The physical body and the etheric body are so intertwined that they are bound together. When one stops functioning, they both stop functioning. Both stop existing after death. The other bodies that function in negative space/time can, possibly, live on after death. What happens at this point is beyond the scope of this book, but both Gerber and Tiller have very specific models that explain concepts of reincarnation and a multidimensional universe that is in line with many esoteric philosophies.

The basic concept here is that the physical body is an instrument of the higher or more subtle bodies. The mind projects an image through the astral body in the form of a hologram to create what we consider our etheric and physical body. In other words, the physical world that modern science is dealing with is a holographic projection in the first place. To understand if that is true or not, we better learn more about holograms and holographic projection.

Holograms

A hologram is actually composed of interference, the crisscrossing of patterns that occur when two or more laser waves meet. Imagine throwing a rock into the clear water of a still pond. You can see the ripples spreading out in expanding concentric circles. Now throw in two rocks, one right after the other, but the second rock several feet away from the first rock. We would start to see the two concentric circles, but after a short time the two circles would meet up with each other. At this point, the pattern ceases to be composed of concentric circles and forms a complex pattern known as interference; that is, the second rock's concentric circle interferes with the first rock's concentric circle.

A wave can create interference with any other like waves, such as sound waves, radio waves or light waves. Lasers are made up of pure, coherent light waves, thus they can create very finely tuned interference patterns. Some have called laser light the perfect pebble and the perfect pond. When we construct interference with laser light, we create a hologram.

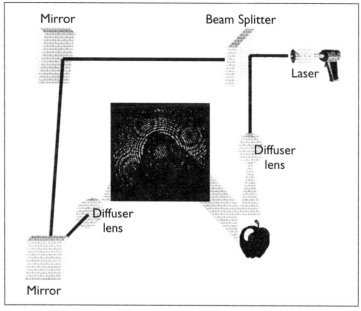

FIGURE **5.5**

A hologram is produced by taking a single beam of laser light and splitting it into two separate beams (see Figure 5.5). The first beam is bounced off an object (say an apple) toward a photographic film. The second beam is allowed to collide with the reflected light from the first beam and together the two beams join to form an interference pattern on the film. To the naked eye, the image on the film is unrecognizable until another laser, or bright light, is shone on it and then a three-dimensional object pops out—in this case an apple. The purer the hologram, the more detailed the image—which appears totally lifelike until touched, then it disappears.

That in itself is remarkable, but the amazing part is that the hologram can be repeatedly broken into many pieces, each of which holds the image of the whole apple. Every time a piece is divided, the hazier the image becomes—which does not detract from the astounding reality that the smallest fragment of the original film contains the same image, and all the information from the whole image.

The Tiller model agrees with many other holistic models, namely that we are holographic projections of our own minds, filtered through the astral body and constructed by the etheric body. The etheric body acts as a blueprint for the DNA to help guide and build the physical body.

Those who study esoterics suggest that the pure light of the laser beam in our universe is the Great Spirit or God. Our mental body (like the apple) is the object that creates the physical body, filtered through the astral and etheric body from an interference pattern. The universal hologram is much more complex than the technology that we have invented to create simple three-dimensional still images. The universal hologram is an ever-moving, animated, changing hologram that folds in upon itself from time to time in order to create what we call reality. Every part of the hologram is connected to every other part. Now this might sound crazy, like some far-out science fiction movie, but it does fit into Eastern cultural models and religious scholarly texts that have been around for millennia.

Briefly, this means that we are an image not only of our mind but also of the universe (built in the image of God), continuously connected and all knowing. The problem seems to be that we are a bit hazy, because we are only a tiny fragment of that existence.

The common esoteric saying, "as above, so below" comes to mind. From the perspective of a hologram, if there is any kind of disorder on any one of the levels of our being, it will have its counterpart on all other levels. This means that specific emotional blocks should show up in the physical body or, conversely, signs in the physical body should help us interpret emotional issues that might be clouding the flow of our higher bodies.

Entrainment

Entrainment is a term in physics wherein two rhythms that have nearly the same frequency become coupled to each other to pattern the same rhythm. Technically, entrainment is mutual phase locking of two (or more) oscillators. For example, several out-of-sync pendulum clocks will eventually entrain, with all of the pendulums swinging in precise synchrony. A human example might be when people who are in agreement with each other walk together (as in holding hands); both right feet go forward at the same time; conversely, if they are in conflict, often their pace will be at odds. Entrainment may be a partial explanation for how birds fly in a flock or fish swim in a school, all in synchronized movement, never bumping into one another.

Entrainment in a group can be a very uplifting phenomena; not to mention entertaining, as when thousands are entraining to a sports team or a musician (which gives us a glimpse of why festivals, mentioned in an earlier chapter, can be so uplifting and releasing). When entrainment represents release it produces a deeper feeling; as it can be positive, negative or neutral, it plays a central role in many aspects of vibrational healing. Here are some specifics on how entrainment works.

Not only are we multidimensional beings (physical, etheric, astral, mental and causal) that share similar electromagnetic frequencies with other humans, all parts of our body are interconnected. If a vibration is sent out and received, it can be felt throughout our being: physical, emotional, mental and causal.

Scientist James Oschman, in his book *Energy Medicine, The Scientific Basis*, puts forward this hypothesis to explain the basis of a vibrational energy approach to the body.

> A complete description of the assembly and operation and repair of a living system requires an understanding of the regulatory effects of both molecules and of energy fields. The genes govern the manufacture of molecules in appropriate quantities, and patterns of forces exerted by energy fields bring molecules together to produce functional structure.

Every part and molecule of the body, as well as the acupuncture meridians of traditional East Asia or Oriental medicine, form a continuously interconnected semiconductor electronic network or organism whose every part is immersed in and generates a constant stream of vibratory information. This is information about all of the activities taking place at any given time throughout the body.

Complete health corresponds to total interconnection. When accumulated physical and/or emotional trauma damages the connection, the body's defense and repair systems become impaired, and disease has a chance to take hold. Acupuncture and other energy therapies restore and balance the vibratory circuitry, with obvious and profound benefits. The body's defense and repair systems are able to repair themselves.

Many individuals, both scientists and therapists, have contributed valuable insights to this emerging picture of how the body functions in health and disease. Phenomena that previously seemed disconnected and unrelated are now complementing one another, giving us a more complete understanding than we would otherwise have.

This vibrational communication system can both heal us or, through the presence of blocks, reduce communication to disconnected areas. A practitioner's goal is to have unblocked communication to all parts. This system works on an energetic level rather than a purely mechanical level. On an individual basis, botanical, homeopathics and flower essences can help entrain us on an energetic level both individually and as a group.

When a group of people focus or entrain to the same concept or focal point, this is also felt through to the cellular and genetic level. These electromagnetic influences also have a profound influence on the other more subtle bodies. Current research even shows that the participants do not have to inhabit the same physical space for entrainment to occur, but can become linked together through common thoughts or goals, such as prayer meetings. This type of entrainment, common attunement or morphic resonance is a profound experience.

Morphic resonance is a concept created by biologist Dr. R. Sheldrake, and it takes place through morphogenetic fields, giving rise to specific structures or behaviors. The notion of a morphogenetic field is another way of talking about the etheric body and its relationship to the physical body. We might use the terms morphic resonance and etheric resonance interchangeably. Organisms tuned in to the same frequency of a morphogenetic field will appear to communicate and learn things almost telepathically. Growth patterns and structure seem to be communicated almost like blueprints through the morphogenetic field. Behavior and structure will be repeated in different organisms, without any other known means of communication except the morphogenetic field. This brings up an interesting concept that was expressed in 1839 by Claude Bernard (father of modern physiology): "the genes create structure, but the genes do not control them; vital force does not create structures, the vital force directs them." This statement reveals what the top medical thinkers were contemplating almost 150 years ago. It also help us understand the magnetic nature of the etheric body.

James Oschman in *Energy Medicine* expresses an almost identical hypothesis:

> A complete description of the assembly and operation and repair of a living system requires an understanding of the regulatory effects of both molecules and of energy fields. The genes govern the manufacture of molecules in appropriate quantities, and patterns of forces exerted by energy fields bring molecules together to produce functional structure.

This model of the body can be compared to the materials used to build a house. Lumber, bricks and mortar will not actually build the house. It takes the life force of the individual tradespeople, following the pattern of the blueprint, to complete the job. The genes will give you either blue or brown "building blocks" to construct the eyes. The vital life energy pattern, directed by the etheric body, creates the blueprint for where the building blocks or eyes will be placed in the body.

When there is injury or disrepair in the body, it is the role of the energy field to direct the healing process (blueprint). If there is miscommunication in the energy field, the building blocks will not be placed in the proper order, thus the repair will not be as functional as in the original plan. The living cellular matrix and crystals provide part of the mechanism for the communication. By using agents such as herbs, acupuncture, healing hands or homeopathy, often essential information is transferred to the tissue to aid in the healing process. This helps fine-tune the process.

It has been shown that an electrical current is generated at an injury site, as some sort of signal that stops once the tissue is completely repaired. This of course signals to the rest of the body that there is an injury, as well as the location and extent of the injury. This, in turn, can attract various white blood cells, fibroblasts and other cells to the wound site. Once the tissue is repaired, the signal stops, giving feedback to the rest of the body. This current has been shown to not be ionic, but a semiconductor current that is sensitive to magnetic fields. The semiconduction takes place in the perineural connective tissue and surrounding parts of the living matrix. This again gives us the impression that the communication is like a circuit board in a computer and that it is the magnetic frequency, perhaps, to which the body responds.

As stated in an earlier chapter, the immune system is like a tuning fork. It reacts in harmony to our environment. If the information of an injury or health issue is communicated properly, the immune system will respond in harmony. If the communication is malfunctioning, then it is not in harmony, thus the immune system will often attack the body instead of the injury—creating autoimmune issues. Botanicals can aid in clearing up the miscommunications through entrainment.

The principle of entrainment also explains how tai chi, yoga and hands-on therapies, such as Rolfing and Heller work, play a role in effecting change at a profound level—because they help the person resonate in harmony with his or her etheric body. This in turn helps communication with all the subtle bodies. By becoming more aware of how we entrain to different vibrational frequencies, we can begin to choose which kind of energy we want to resonate with and decide whether that is healing for us.

The heart and health

We now know that the heart plays a unique and hitherto unrecognized role in balancing the whole human system and that it is also an endocrine gland that secretes hormones to balance the cardiovascular system. The heart possesses its own nervous system and magnetic properties, all of which function independently of the central nervous system (CNS). The rhythm of the heartbeat entrains various other organs and systems, including the immune system and the brain. The emotional states—both positive and negative—have been shown to dramatically affect the electrical rhythms generated by the heart, thus affecting the rest of the body. Negative emotional states have proved to be immunosuppressive and positive emotions to be immunostimulative. Therefore, it would seem that energy generated by the heart can impact immunity.

The heart is the largest producer of rhythmic energy in the body, both electrically and mechanically. It produces 50 times more electrical energy and 1,000 times more electromagnetic energy than the brain. This electromagnetic energy is not confined to the body, being measurable several feet away. This electromagnetic energy, along with the electromagnetic energy of the chakra system, constitute another communication system that is fluid with the psychoneuroimmunology (PNI) communication system.

The Heart Chakra is a Center of Entrainment

In the chakra system, the heart is the halfway point in the body; three centers are below and three above. The heart center represents lessons about giving and receiving love and about transcending individual ego. Lessons of the heart are commonly about loss, grief, suffering and separation from those we love. As a result, we learn not only the power of love but also compassion for the suffering of others. Health issues connected to the heart center usually reflect emotional concerns of this nature. While physically a change in diet is needed to reduce cholesterol, meditation on the nature of personal relationships is also necessary. It is little wonder that most health issues are alleviated or improved when the patient has positive emotional relationships in his or her life. Those who feel isolated, lonely or without love have far more difficulty recovering from illnesses. Even having a pet has been shown to have a very positive effect on the immune system. A recent study has shown that on average, spending three to five minutes daily with a cat or dog, can have a more positive effect on the immune system than spending hours with a spouse! Interestingly, many religious and esoteric groups feel that the love of the heart can heal all.

The magnetic property already mentioned might be directly influenced by energy from the fourth (heart) chakra. Entrainment from the other bodies seems to be especially important to set the rhythm of the heart, and therefore the rest of the physical body. As Myss says, "The fourth chakra is the central powerhouse of the human energy system. The middle chakra, it mediates between the body and spirit and determines their health. Fourth chakra energy is emotional in nature and helps propel our emotional development."

A healthy fourth chakra is one of the keys to a healthy immune system in the physical body.

SUMMARY POINTS

1. The William Tiller model shows that there is an explanatory model for the subtle bodies.

2. Through Einstein's famous equation ($E=mc^2$) we can see that kinetic energy increases to near infinite as we approach the speed of light. Thus traditional physicists think that nothing can go faster than the speed of light.

3. Using the square root of negative numbers (e.g., -2) we get a set of imaginary numbers that mathematician Charles Muses calls hypernumbers; these, he believes, describe higher-dimension phenomena such as the subtle bodies.

4. Entropy describes the tendency toward disorder. Negative entropy describes the tendency toward order. Vital energy appears to be negative entropy.

5. The subtle bodies take up negative space, but positive time. This would make the subtle bodies magnoelectric, instead of electromagnetic.

6. The chakras reside at the etheric level of being, the interface between the emotional body and the physical body. They are of an electrostatic nature, most likely comprising magnoelectric energy.

7. Many therapeutic agents such as herbs, flower essences and homeopathy deliver some of the healing properties via the energetic of their subtle bodies.

8. Tiller describes three separate mental bodies representing instinctive function, intellectual function and low spiritual function.

9. The emotional body is the containment body, which represents a holographic projection of the mental bodies.

10. Holograms are made by the interference patterns of pure laser light, reflected off an object.

11. Universal energy is reflected from our mental body to form the holographic image of our physical body: "as above, so below."

12. Entrainment occurs when two rhythms or similar frequencies couple to each other.

13. All the parts of our body are connected in a continuously flowing communication system. Blocks in that communication system can cause disease.

14. Physiologist Claude Bernard states, "The genes create structure, but the genes do not control them: vital force does not create structure, the vital force directs them."

15. The heart, as well as the fourth chakra heart center, can help balance the whole system, both physically and emotionally.

PART THREE

The Treatment Processes

CHAPTER SIX

Plant Alchemy:
Plants as Teachers

❧

I was first introduced to plants as teachers by an Indian medicine man back in the early 1970s. After finishing my first degree (in environmental biology), and urged by one of my professors, I decided to write a book about the edible and medicinal plants of my local area. How to do this? Well, experience it firsthand and become one with it, of course. So I gathered together what few resources I had, bought a tepee and moved into the mountains. This was the only way to access the material for that book.

That summer was so enjoyable that I decided to be daring and try living in the mountains year-round. Could I make it through the winter living in a tepee? After all, in these locations temperatures could easily plummet to −45°F. Well, if people had done so for thousands of years, so could I. However, trying to survive by myself would be stupid, so I looked for a like-minded group of people who were experienced in winter outdoor living and was lucky enough to find a group that included some Indian medicine men. I joined them with the idea of furthering my knowledge of herbal medicines. That winter I started my herbal apprenticeship in the First Nation tradition. (Aboriginal people in Canada refer to themselves as First Nation peoples.)

I remember those first days sitting in front of Buffalo Child, one of my new mentors. I asked, "If all these herbs had such strong medicinal properties and could cure so many diseases, where was the book about it? Where could I read the proof?" I was still clinging to my academic hat. I wanted some printed literature to assure me I was on the right trail. He looked at me and said, "Well it is written down, boy. It is written in the way the wind blows through the pines; the way the creek flows, the coyote howls and the rocks lie; and when you can learn to read, you'll be a herbalist."

Whew! I didn't know I was going to get in that deep! I had so much to learn, and unlearn, since my biology training. I began to see through my mentor's eyes that all things are alive; not only the plants but also rocks, the entire planet we live on and the energies that flow through it. The role of a Native healer is to match the energies of a person with the corresponding treatment. Therefore, if someone is deficient in a certain energy, the healer tries to find that missing energy from the environment: maybe with a herb, an exercise, a story or a ritual. Trickery is also a perfectly acceptable means of changing a person's energies. Interestingly, many Indian languages do not have a precise word for medicine man—often the translation more closely resembles the idea of a trickster.

As apprentices, our task was to learn the personality of the medicinal plant and other substances in our environment. We had to learn the plant's story: this was done by spending long periods with the plant to understand and be aware of its energies or by listening to stories told by the elders and medicine people. One of my favorite stories was that of the now-endangered species, lady's slipper.

A lady's-slipper legend

There was once a young daughter of an Indian chieftain. One day, while she was playing far away from her camp she came across a baby rabbit. The rabbit was crying. He had hurt his feet and couldn't go home and feared his mother would be angry with him. The little girl begged the rabbit to stop crying and gave him her moccasins, so he could travel home without further damaging his feet.

It was growing late and the child decided to return to her camp. It wasn't long before she realized why the little rabbit had cut his feet. The trail was full of very sharp stones and her feet were now torn and bleeding. Exhausted, she collapsed along the wooded pathway and fell asleep. Before long a songbird flew by and, seeing her bleeding feet, begged the Great Spirit to help the poor little maiden. On awakening, she found a beautiful pair of moccasins hanging on two slender stems. She slipped these moccasins on her bleeding feet and was able to make her way home.

If you don't believe this story, look inside a yellow lady's-slipper orchid; you'll find the reddish purple spots of blood and some lines made by the little maiden's bleeding feet.

This story reveals the many dimensions of a wonderful herb. First, the character of the young but aristocratic maiden imparts a quality of gentleness and strength. The little crying rabbit illustrates the sad emotions that the herb can treat. The concept of injury shows that this is a superior herb for easing pain, often lulling a person into a gentle sleep when they are distressed. Finally, the herb will protect from pain and irritation, so we can find our way "home."

Such tales teach us about the different aspects of the elements found all around us. We are reminded that each plant or creature has its own story and its own vibration.

Biolife is negative entropy

Negative entropy is the force that aids in building and organizing life, as opposed to positive entropy, the process of decay. Negative entropy is a part of what makes the physical body take on a "life force" and is integral to the process of biolife. All biological life on this planet must possess or be guided by negative entropy. Since all organisms have biolife, they would also have more subtle bodies in addition to their physical body. Hence, a medicinal plant substance, like all biolife, is composed of more than just a physical body. The plant's story or personality indicates the composition of its subtle bodies. It is possible for us to access this subtle plant body material to create healing.

Botanicals also have a life: plant energetics

Botanicals have subtle bodies, and we can work with their subtle body energy for healing. Even though they have their own vibrational frequencies that respond to the plant kingdom, for the sake of this discussion we will represent these subtle bodies as the emotional and mental components of the plants.

There are many people in diverse cultures who have described these more subtle aspects or energetics of the plant kingdom. They are portrayed as hot or cold, sweet or sour, ascending or descending, yin or yang, and relaxant or stimulant; many other energetic terms can be found in the lexicon of, among others, Oriental, ancient Greek and Indian medicine. Universally, most practitioners using botanical remedies use them from an energetic perspective.

I often consider plants to be as much teachers as medicinal substances. How do we know in what form to use a herb or which preparations will communicate with our different bodies? The healer's purpose is to match the right botanical preparation's energetics to the individual's subtle bodies or energy field. Different forms of plant preparations tend to show stronger action on a specific body.

Doctrine of signature

A live plant, growing in a field or garden, contains all of its own attributes: physical, emotional, mental and its own connection to the universal hologram. In fact, we could say, like us, plants' physical representation is at least partly a projection of these attributes, of their particular holographic reality. The visual appearance of plants often reflects their energetics. Many ancient healers called this the "doctrine of signatures." For example, a heart-shaped leaf was considered good for the heart—sometimes only the leaf was used, other times, the whole plant. When an entire living plant is used, all its attributes are accessed, which is why some herbalists prefer to make live plant extracts, feeling this captures the full essence of the botanical.

Physical body

The next stage in processing a plant or herb is to dry the whole plant—or one of its parts—and use that. The dried plant can then be used as a capsule, tablet or further processed into a tea, tincture or fluid extract. Here, we also get attributes of the whole plant (physical and subtle body energetics), but we are concentrating more on the physical qualities. This simple broad-based spectrum is the most common method of preparation in North America, and provides easy-to-use dosage. Crude herbs (dried unprocessed plant material) are particularly good if the specific chemicals or "active ingredients" of a botanical are required. For example, if extracting the phytosterol function of black cohosh (*Cimifuga*) or if the vitamin C from an orange is needed, this crude or standardized extract is the best. When a specific amount of a particular chemical is wanted, the botanical is more than a good delivery system. In addition to the chemical, the vital energy (qi) and the personality of the herb are also delivered. Instead of getting a pizza from a store, it's like having a good friend deliver the pizza then stay for some mutually enjoyable conversation and socializing.

If the full function of a plant is required—for its physical attributes (physiological dosing)—it is best to use a simple dried form of the herb (usually found in tablets or capsules). If a specific amount of a certain chemical is desired, a standardized or guaranteed potency extract is best.

Etheric body

There is a tradition in herbal medicine that goes back to the ancients and was also much used by the American eclectic John M. Scudder, MD in the latter part of the nineteenth and early part of the twentieth century. This tradition is used today by contemporary herbalists like Matthew Wood, and is called a "simple."

Simples are often used in 1–3 drop doses (instead of 20–60 drops for physiological effect). After a person receives a specific diagnosis, a specific remedy is given at this drop level. You can learn more about this in *The Book of Herbal Wisdom* by Matthew Wood or *Specific Medication* by Scudder. In these cases the energetic of the herb is as important, if not more so, than its physical attributes. I consider this drop level to be working more on the level of the etheric body. The single herb–single drop remedies can produce a strong and profound movement on a health issue. It is tempting to think more is stronger, or "bigger is better," but if you get the right botanical with the right energetic for the problem, the single-drop remedies are much more profound with better healing action. They achieve the healing action through entrainment. The botanical remedy sets up a "pattern" or "blueprint" that "teaches" the etheric bodies vital energy patterns. This in turn sets up a new flow of energy that can be used to heal the whole system.

Astral or emotional body

The next of our bodies is the astral body. The emotional body can be affected quite well by using a whole crude herb, but if you feel the problem is primarily emotional in nature, you are better off to use a flower essence, such as Bach flower remedies, California Essence or the likes. This form of botanical works specifically on emotions. They are chosen for the emotional situation of the person, not the physical attribute. This is not to say that these remedies don't help the physical problem, *au contraire*. Let's say a person is immobilized by an inability to make decisions, preventing them from moving forward in their life. He or she also shows signs of arthritis. If the center of gravity of the health issue was the emotional immobility, he or she should take the Bach flower remedy Scleranthus, ignoring the physical issue of arthritis. This should release the issue of emotional immobility and produce significant changes in the arthritis too, often to the degree of ridding the body of all symptoms. In this case, the emotion of immobility was causing the arthritis. We will look at how these remedies are made in a moment, but suffice it to say that they are much more subtle than the crude herb or the single-drop dosage form of the herb.

Mental body

If the issue is a combination of emotional and mental, we would use homeopathic remedies rather than the other dosage form. Even though the decision making on which homeopathic remedy is used is done for physical, emotional and mental attributes, the energy of the homeopathic remedy treats the more subtle vibrations of our higher frequency bodies, which in turn makes changes in the physical body. Some problems are miasms or blocks (we will explain these shortly) that originate from ancestral issues and/or a particular personality type or life experiences. The vibrational frequency, or subtle body of the person taking the remedy, depends on the potency of the remedy. We will find out more about potency when we see how it is made.

1. Live or fresh plant extract—all bodies, with equally distributed concentration.
2. Crude herb—all bodies, but stronger concentration on the physical body.
3. Standardized extract—specific physical biochemical processes.
4. Single-drop specifics—etheric body.
5. Flower essence—astral or emotional body.
6. Homeopathic—mostly mental but also astral, etheric and physical depending on potency.

To recap, even though each form of botanical remedy has a specific center of gravity for one of the bodies, all remedies work on all bodies to a degree.

Making the remedies

All of the preparation can usually be bought in a health food store or from a herbalist. The following are methods of preparation to illustrate how they function at a more subtle vibrational level and in case you would like to try and make them yourself.

Plant Extracts

For a standard dried herb tincture:

Ingredients to make a 1 in 5 (1:5) tincture

- 100 g amount of herb
- 500 g amount of 40 percent grain alcohol

Method

- Soak the herb in the alcohol and shake every few days for two weeks
- Drain off the tincture
- Press the remaining herb mass (marc) with a press (for example, a hydraulic one) to extract as much liquid as possible.

Variations

— To make a fluid extract (which is more concentrated than a tincture), use a greater botanical to alcohol ratio: possibly one to one.

— To make a more concentrated extract, allow for some evaporation (usually over moderate heat as in a double boiler) until the desired concentration is obtained.

The 1:5 tincture is the most common type to be found in the marketplace. Fluid extracts are 1:4, 1:2 or even 1:1. Unless otherwise stated, the product is most likely a standard 1:5 tincture.

Fresh plant extracts are made in a similar way, but instead use fresh plant rather than dried plant material. There is an elaborate formula to compensate for the water content of the herb to adjust the percentage of alcohol.

The use of crude herbs in the form of tea, capsules or tablets is quite straightforward. From either the tincture, fluid extract or the fresh plant extract, a practitioner would choose the single-drop remedy, depending on which tradition he or she follows.

Flower essences and the sunshine method

While most people will choose to buy a prepared flower essence, understanding the key to how they are made will provide a better appreciation of their vibrational energy. The most common way to prepare flower essence remedies is the sunshine method: a thin, glass bowl is filled with the purest water available (spring water, not distilled, is best). Immediately after picking, the plant's blooms are floated on the water so that they cover the entire surface. Then, the bowl is left in the sunshine for three to four hours, or for less time should the blooms show signs of fading. The blossoms are then carefully lifted out and the water is poured into bottles, filling them halfway; the remaining half is filled with brandy to preserve the resulting remedies. This is called the mother tincture.

Administering the dose of flower essence

From the mother tincture take two to four drops and put them in another bottle filled with equal parts of brandy and spring water and potentized (pounded approximately 100 times on the counter). This bottle is referred to as the "stock bottle."

Put two or three drops from the stock bottle into a one-ounce bottle that is not quite filled with pure water. If you need to keep the remedy some time (more than a week), 50% brandy (40 percent alcohol—80 proof) should be added as a preservative. From this last bottle a few drops should be taken straight into the mouth or in a little water or juice. As you can see, flower essences are very, very dilute extracts of the flower. They really don't have any chemical content but contain vibrational content instead.

The use of flower essence is symptom related. If the corresponding emotion is strong and reoccurring, the essence may be given every few minutes until an improvement is noticed; in less dramatic cases, every half hour and, in long-standing cases, every two to three hours. Moderate cases are dosed once or twice a day. Moisten the lips frequently with the remedy for people who are unconscious. Flower essences can be added to lotions and washes when desired.

As explained, these remedies rely completely on the vibrational level (or life force) of the plant, not the chemical nature of the herb. The effect of flower essences is similar to the effect of listening to a powerful, moving piece of music. The sound waves reach your ears, but the results effect your emotions, right through to your soul. Music can also affect breathing, pulse rate and other physical systems. The flower essences are considered to be a specific pattern of the holographic matrix of the originating plant, which directly affects our emotions, rather than the physical body. Edward Bach, the founder of flower essence therapy stated, "they flood our nature with the particular virtue we need, and wash out from us the fault that is causing the harm." Contemporary researchers, like Patricia Kaminski and Richard Katz, authors of *Flower Essence Repertory*, feel that flower essences work on an alchemical law of polarities called the Union of Opposites, by which polar opposites are integrated into higher vibrations.

The book I most use in this area is *Flower Essence Repertory*, which cross-references more than 300 emotions and lists the particular emotional nuance as it relates to the specific flower essences. A few are:

- Devitalization
- Habit patterns
- Immune disturbances
- Perfectionism
- Sensitivity
- Vitality

I have found the following remedies to be most pertinent to autoimmune-type problems. At the end of the book, in the Repertory section, you will find more remedies for each of several autoimmune health conditions.

Devitalization

Even though there are sixteen remedies listed under devitalization, we will look at the eleven that I most commonly use.

Garlic—lack of vitality due to fear, nervousness or parasitic entities

Hibiscus—loss of sexual responsiveness; inability to experience sexuality as an expression of soul warmth

Morning glory—low energy from destructive habits; addictions

Nasturtium—tendency toward dry intellectualism; lack of life force

Nicotiana—mechanization of body, tendency to see the body as a machine; suppression of emotions, leading to reduced life forces or vitality

Olive—depletion of physical vitality after a long illness or struggle

Pink yarrow—feeling drained of energy from absorbing the negative emotions of others

Rosemary—lack of physical warmth and presence; cold extremities and poor circulation

St. John's wort—living too much at the periphery of consciousness; expanded state of consciousness that drains vital forces

Yarrow—feeling drained of energy due to harsh environment or the negative/hostile thoughts of others

Zinnia—tendency toward overseriousness; feeling dull and lifeless

Habit Patterns

Cayenne—breaking free of habitual behavior; fiery catalyst for change

Chestnut bud—constant repetition of experiences without learning from them; attachment to habit patterns that are regressive and limiting

Morning glory—to overcome destructive habits; to develop lifestyle patterns based upon health rhythms

Rock water—holding overly strict and unyielding habit patterns based upon extreme ideals of discipline and control

Sagebrush—breaking free of old identities and habits that are no longer appropriate; finding what is essential or true for oneself

Walnut—letting go of habits or lifestyle patterns taken on from the influence of others

Immune Disturbances

Beech—overidentification with exterior surroundings, leading to sensitive, reactive or critical behavior and immune dysfunction

Crab apple—oversensitivity and obsession with impurity, leading to reduced ability to tolerate toxins; hyperallergic

Echinacea—maintaining the integrity and essential nature of self despite circumstances of degradation, abuse or environmental assault; for compromised immune system

Garlic—attraction to lower psychic phenomena, opening oneself physically and psychically to parasitic entities

Lavender—hypersensitivity leading to nervous exhaustion and related stress to immune system

Love-lies-bleeding—to increase immune response by finding meaning in one's illness or disease; to shift from victim to participant in healing process

Morning glory—compromised immunity due to damaged etheric body; need to rebuild rhythmic connection to nature and etheric body

Nasturtium—lowered vitality and immunity due to overly intellectual lifestyle

Olive—extreme fatigue and exhaustion; depletion of defenses, both physical and psychic

Self-heal—Strengthening health-creating forces; self-responsibility as a pathway to self-healing

Walnut—following convictions; creating inner strength and integrity of self

Yarrow—oversensitivity to social or physical environment; absorption of psychic or physical toxins, leading to fatigue and depletion

Yarrow special formula—vulnerability to negative energies and substances in the environment, such as radiation, electro-magnetic fields, allergens, pollution

Perfectionism

There are twenty-seven remedies available; here are seven.

Beech—tendency to blame and criticize others due to high standards of perfectionism

Chamomile—becoming easily upset; difficulty dealing with challenging emotions or strife

Dandelion—overplanning; enslaving the body to impossible standards of performance

Fiaree—obsession with details disproportionate to their real importance; draining energy through worry and over-concern

Pine—inability to forgive oneself for errors; self-deprecation when performance is less than perfect

Scarlet monkeyflower—repressing core levels of anger and rage in order to appear "nice"

Willow—blaming others for adverse situations; inability to accept and let go

Sensitivity

There are twenty-five remedies available; here are six.

Aspen—hypersensitive to things unseen or unknown; need for psychic balance

Beech—oversensitive to others and the environment, leading to hypercritical nature; blaming others for one's own suffering

Nicotiana—inability to cope with sensitivity, compulsion to numb or deaden the soul's experience

Pink yarrow—oversensitivity to emotions of others and internalizing their problems

Red chestnut—overconcern about the problems of others; fear and worry

St. John's wort—overexpanded psyche; vulnerability to harmful influences

Vitality

There are fifteen remedies available; here are six.

Aloe vera—to restore life force and replenish the heart center; especially for feeling burned out from too much "fire"

Arnica—repairing life energy after shock or trauma

Lady's-slipper—nervous exhaustion and sexual depletion

Mountain pennyroyal—clear, vital thinking, especially when threatened by the thoughts and energies absorbed from others

Nasturtium—overly dry intellectualism; needing more earthy vitality

Wild rose—rallying life forces to fight a long illness; overcoming a tendency to apathy and resignation

The above emotions often apply to those suffering from chronic fatigue syndrome and fibromyalgia. Again, it is important to remember that we are looking at the emotions, not the physical symptoms, but these are the types of emotions that are associated with this group of disorders.

It is normal to use only up to five ingredients at a time. Only one essence may apply, but if needed you can put up to five essences in a remedy. Once it has been decided which are the most important remedies, take a few drops from the stock bottle and add them to a one-ounce bottle of water with about 1/3 brandy in it. Often a review of the emotion is done in one to three weeks to find several of the emotions are reduced or have disappeared. At this time, the remedies might be changed to include others that now seem more important. The good news is that flower essences have no side effects and no drug interactions as there is no chemistry involved. They are vibrations. If the astral body is not tuned to their frequency, they will not be picked up, similar to how you pick up only the radio station you tune to on a radio. If a person takes the wrong remedy, it will just not have an effect on him or her, as he or she is not tuned in to it.

You can easily buy stock remedies in health food stores and make up remedies that you feel are most appropriate for you.

Flower essence shorts

People are continually testing new flower remedies, adding to the existing stable of essences. Because autoimmune disorders generally include a significant emotional component, I use a lot of flower essence in the treatment of these disorders. Here are the flower remedies most often associated with the emotional profiles of autoimmune patients. Again, this is not an exhaustive list, it is merely a sampling.

Beech (*Fagus sylvatica*)

*   Positive qualities: tolerance, acceptance of others' differences and imperfections, seeing the good within each person and situation

- Patterns of imbalance: judgmental, critical, intolerant, perfectionist, overly sensitive to physical and social environment

Assists those who tend to be overly critical of others; feel inferior, vulnerable or insecure, because they often grew up in an environment of criticism and harsh expectations that in turn makes them hypersensitive to both the physical and psychic environment, and intolerant of imperfections in others.

Chamomile (*Matricaria recutita*)

- Positive qualities: emotional balance, serenity, sunny disposition
- Pattern of imbalance: difficulty releasing emotional tension, easily upset, moody and irritable

Unlike a steady sunny day, people who can use chamomile are moody and subject to ever-fluctuating emotions. They tend to accumulate psychic tension during the day (especially in the stomach), and have a hard time releasing even in dreams, thus often experiencing insomnia. Chamomile aids in releasing tension in the stomach and solar plexus area.

Chaparral (*Larrea tridentata*)

- Positive qualities: a deep penetrating understanding of the transpersonal aspect of self, with a balanced psychic awareness
- Pattern of imbalance: chaotic inner life, disturbed dreams, physically and psychically toxic; drug addiction

Chaparral is a great physical and psychic cleanser, especially when the dream state is chaotic, and is indicated when a person has been overexposed to violent or disturbing images. It is beneficial for detoxifying drugs, especially psychiatric drugs. Chaparral is useful if a person has too much astral debris.

Elm *(Ulmus procera)*

- Positive qualities: confidence and faith to complete tasks; joyous service
- Pattern of imbalance: overwhelmed by the duties and responsibilities of the task

Feeling overwhelmed by a task often emerges from a level of perfectionism, unrealistic goals, and overestimating of what should be achieved. The elm person often builds the importance of the task up so high that he or she feels he or she can't complete it.

Evening Primrose *(Oenothera hookeri)*

- Positive qualities: form deep committed relations because of the ability to open up emotionally; being both aware and capable of healing early negative emotions absorbed from the mother
- Pattern of imbalance: feeling rejected and unwanted; difficulty with commitment in relationship; emotional and sexual repression

This flower helps those who have absorbed strong emotion from their parents, especially the mother either in the womb or as an infant; and who carry a feeling of rejection from this stage and therefore have a hard time making emotional commitments. They will avoid emotional contact or bonding, especially sexually.

Golden Ear Drop *(Dicentra chrysantha)*

- Positive qualities: releasing painful emotional memories of the past, getting a feeling of well-being from childhood experiences

- Pattern of imbalance: have strong emotional tie to painful emotions of the past; suppressed negative emotions of childhood

Due to traumatic periods in their childhood, these individuals often have emotional amnesia as a survival mechanism. This essence helps memory and cleanses the emotions, especially heart energy—often by producing tears—and assists in turning an earlier trauma into a positive strength.

Nicotiana (*Nicotiana alata*)

- Positive qualities: integration of physical and emotional well-being through harmonious connection with Earth energy; deep heart-centered peace
- Pattern of imbalance: numbing the emotions by hardening the body; inability to cope with deep feelings and finer sensibilities

The numbing of emotion occurs when individuals are hardened to the physical and psychic environment. This essence will help bring peace and a sense of connection with life. Useful for tobacco or other addictions, especially when the addiction makes the person feels separate from the true world he or she lives in.

Oak (*Quercus robur*)

- Positive qualities: balanced strength, knowing when to surrender and accept limitations
- Pattern of imbalance: striving beyond one's limits, iron-willed and inflexible

This essence is used when an individual is already strong but is always testing that strength to and beyond its limits.

Consequently, the individual is often too rigid and prone to feelings of superiority. This remedy helps with the surrender to and acceptance of limitations.

Olive (*Olea europaea*)

- Positive qualities: revitalization through connection with the inner self
- Pattern of imbalance: deep exhaustion after a long ordeal

Olive will relieve extreme physical exhaustion for those who are usually overidentified with the physical world. This remedy will help them gain strength by opening up to their own more subtle energies as a source of revitalization and understand that the physical body is connected to higher states of consciousness.

Pink Monkeyflower (*Mimulus lewisii*)

- Positive qualities: courage to take emotional risks; emotional openness and honesty
- Pattern of imbalance: fear of rejection and exposure; feelings of guilt, unworthiness and shame; masking feelings from others and self

The fear of being exposed is very common among autoimmune patients who do not want to reveal their pain and vulnerability. They are very good at constructing masks to hide deeply internalized wounds from the past. These highly sensitive people usually want to reach out and touch others, but usually fail to make real contact. This remedy aids in opening the heart and helping a person realize that by opening up and risking vulnerability he or she can experience the warmth of human love and affection.

Pink Yarrow (*Achillea millefolium*)

- Positive qualities: loving awareness of others from self-contained consciousness; appropriate emotional boundaries
- Pattern of imbalance: influenced by negative forces, overly absorbent auric field, lack of emotional clarity, dysfunctional merging with others

This individual needs to set firm boundaries between self and other, and will likely be "allergic" to emotional confusion due to extreme sensitivity.

Sagebrush (*Artemisia tridentata*)

- Positive qualities: capable of transformation and change due to a deep awareness of inner self
- Pattern of imbalance: need to purify the self to release dysfunctional aspects of personality and surroundings; overly identified with own persona and physical environment

When people are too attached to ego and material possessions, they have a hard time obtaining the detachment needed to contact higher aspects of the self. Sagebrush assists in making contact with the true self, which produces a feeling of spiritual freedom and release.

Yarrow (*Achillea millefolium*)

- Positive qualities: inner radiance and strength of aura, compassionate awareness, inclusive sensitivity, beneficent healing forces
- Pattern of imbalance: extreme vulnerability to others and to environment, easily depleted, overly absorbent of negative influences and psychic toxicity

Today, those on a spiritual path, like their forebears, need that same protection from the outside world while still maintaining daily roles in modern society. Yarrow will help this process as it helps heal "leaky auras" for sensitive people. A Yarrow formula is considered by many as a protection from radiation for cancer treatment.

Yerba Santa (*Eriodictyon californicum*)

- Positive qualities: free-flowing emotions, able to express the range of human emotions from joy and bliss to pain and sadness
- Pattern of imbalance: constricted feeling, especially in the chest; internalization of grief and melancholy with deeply repressed emotions.

The "holy herb" addresses the inner sanctity of the soul, which often gets cluttered with vulnerable emotions of sadness and grief. Yerba santa helps bring these emotions to consciousness, so they can be dealt with and released.

Homeopathy

I remember once seeing an advertisement that posed the question: What do Tina Turner, Mother Teresa and Queen Elizabeth II all have in common? The answer is, they all relied on homeopathic remedies as their major form of health care.

Around the world, homeopathy is one of the major forms of medicinal treatments, and is currently enjoying a renaissance in North America. In the late 1800s and early 1900s, a significant percentage of American hospitals and schools used homeopathy. The discovery of modern homeopathy is credited to the German physician, Samuel Hahnemann (1755–1843), who created cures based on the concept of "like cures like." There is suitable evidence that others, such as the great alchemist Paracelsus (1493–1541), used homeopathic principles, as well as Oriental applications of these principles.

A contemporary example: cutting onions. Tears, runny nose and burning eyes are all likely effects of either cutting onions or being near someone who is cutting them. This is a simple proving. A homeopath would take the evidence of that proving and use the onion for those who have burning, tearful eyes and running noses, because they represent the homeopathic picture of onions. The homeopath gives a very dilute dosage of the onion; in fact, the more minute the dosage, the stronger the remedy.

Making homeopathic remedies

To make a homeopathic remedy you take one part of the tincture (also referred to as the "mother") and add it to nine parts water

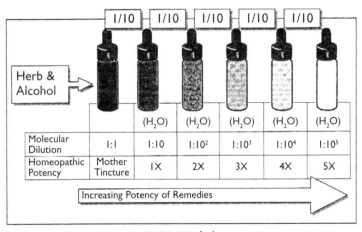

FIGURE **6.1**

alcohol mixture, potentize it by succussion (pounding the bottle of the mixture on the counter approximately 100 times). This becomes 1x (see Figure 6.1). From the 1x you take one part and add it to nine parts water alcohol and potentize it to get 2x. This procedure is done until you get the desired strength. Low-potency homeopathics are between 6x and 12x, or 10^{-6} and 10^{-12}. Medium potency is in the 30x (10^{-30}) range and high potency is over 100x (10^{-100}). The "x," or in some parts of Europe "d," represents a one in ten based on the decimal system. Some homeopaths use a one part in ninety-nine method, designated by a "C," with succussions at each step; so a 5 C is 10^{-10}. This would be similar to 10x, but not quite the same, as it has half as many succussions. It should be pointed out that a law of chemistry (Avogadro's constant) says that after a substance is diluted past 10^{-23} there are no molecules from the original substance in the solution.

The more diluted the remedy, the stronger it is from a homeopathic perspective.

How do homeopathic remedies work?

The theory of water memory—which also applies to flower essences—is a personal favorite. A simple analogy for this theory is the old-fashioned sun print. Placing a plant on photosensitive paper, covering it and leaving it in the sun, and then developing it photochemically, produces the imprint of the plant on the photographic paper (the shadow of the plant). In the case of homeopathic remedies, we get the imprint of the plant on water. In the now-famous paper by Davenas, Benveniste, Poitevin, et al (*Nature*, June 1988) they present the theory that homeopathic substances imprint their vibrational frequency on water. This imprint is most likely held in the angle of the hydrogen to the

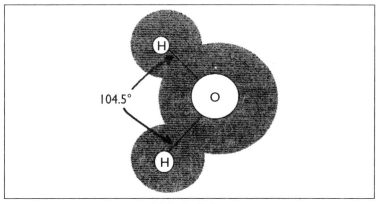

FIGURE **6.2**

oxygen molecule. Instead of the angle being the typical 104.5°, slight variation in that angle (see Figure 6.2) acts like a tuning fork to resonate the frequency of the homeopathic substance.

Since the human body is made up more from water than any other substance, it is understandable that the electromagnetic frequency in both flower essences and homeopathics can trigger a "reaction" or an entrainment in the body.

Again, the higher the dilution, the more potent the homeopathic. The lower potencies, 6x to 12x, deal more with current issues occurring in the physical body. For example, a hand recently injured from being slammed in a car door could be treated with arnica 6x to 12x, which would be very effective for reducing pain, bruising and swelling, and speeding up the healing process. However, if the injury was a few week or months old, arnica 30x would be more effective to rid the body of trauma associated with the accident; and for an accident or trauma that is years old, arnica 100x or 10C would be better. The greater the potency, the further back it will go in fixing the incident and the higher in the vibrational spectrum it will go in the individual taking it. The treatment of emotional issues requires at least 30x if not higher; likely 100x. If the situation is more associated with the mental body, 1M (M=1000x) or higher would be suitable. The more potent the homeopathic, the more subtle the energy it can work on.

Miasms

Another important concept in homeopathy is "miasm." Hahnemann often found that even though he felt he had the right remedy, and the patient responded well for a while, relapse would occur. After studying this group of people, he noticed they all had similar blocks. He suspected that these features had caused blocks to the action of the remedy. He called these blocks "miasms" and created a comprehensive theory around them. The important thing to do was to get rid of the miasm before going on to other remedies. Hahnemann defined three miasms: "psora" which was associated with skin disease; "sycosis" associated with suppressed gonorrhea; and "syphilis" associated with suppressed syphilis. Many home-opaths have developed others, including cancer, as a combination of several miasms. When a homeopath encounters a miasmatic block in a patient, it has to be cleared before proceeding. One interesting aspect of miasms is that they need not occur in an individual's lifetime in order to have an effect on that person. For example, your great grandfather might have suppressed the symptoms of syphilis by using a pharmaceutical like mercury, and it may still affect you.

The concept of miasm has also been adopted by other disci-plines. For example, some psychologists suggest that early childhood trauma or post-traumatic stress syndrome is a type of mias-matic block (trapped emotions due to the trauma) that has to be cleared before other healing work can be done.

Consequently, the idea is to first identify where the center of gravity of the health issue is located. Is it more physical, etheric, emotional or mental? Often the disorder has a center of gravity in more than one place or it is hard to identify the area on which to focus, so a combination of remedies is used. A person might take something for a structural issue and his or her immune system in crude herb form, a flower essence to deal with emotional issues and even a homeopathic, all at the same time.

SUMMARY POINTS

1. Like us, plants have subtle bodies.
2. The doctrine of signatures explains that sometimes the shape of the plant will help us determine the energetics of a plant.
3. Medicinal plants are much more than a delivery system for chemicals. Their energetic represents a "personality" that can influence our subtle bodies and physical body.
4. Standardized or guaranteed potency herbs are good to use when a specific amount of chemical for a exact biochem-ical process is required.
5. Single-drop specifics are good when dealing with the etheric body.
6. Flower essences are best for healing on the astral or emotional body.
7. Homeopathic remedies work on the emotional and mental aspects of our being.

8. Homeopathic frequencies are held in the memory of water.

9. Miasms are energy blocks that stop other therapeutic remedies from working.

10. It is important to determine the center of gravity of the health issue before deciding on the best remedy. Is it more physical, emotional or mental in nature?

Herbs
as Teachers

During my years as a practicing herbalist, I have learned to respect many of the botanicals that I use more as teachers than just medicinal tools. The number of herbs that could be catalogued here is substantial so I have restrained myself by listing selected favorites and the most valuable herbs for dealing with autoimmune and stress-related problems. Keeping with the format of this book, we have not included scientific references for these herbs. We have listed books that we found useful in gathering this information at the end of the book. For those who want a more detailed reference for these herbs, you can get that information at our Web site: www.wildrosecollege.com and go to the *materia medica* tab. You can also look at the Web site: www.mind-bodyharmony.com.

The herbs that we are going to describe here are:

Reishi
St. John's wort
Kava kava
Skullcap
Siberian ginseng
Red root
Barberry

These herbs are from the plant and fungus kingdoms. Each has its own personality and strength, as well as much to teach.

Please note: The following information is not intended to be used as a substitution for consultation with your physician or health care practitioner.

Reishi: the wise counselor

The year was 1996. I had filled a number of busy years crisscrossing North America, given lectures on plant medicine, answered questions on innumerable radio shows and chased down rare books for my own research. Consequently, hundreds of thousands of frequent flyer points had accumulated and now it was time to cash some in. Since my work entailed so much travel, I was not able to spend as much time as I wanted with my teenage kids. So once every few years, I enjoyed offering each of my children the opportunity to take an adventure trip with me. This time it was my daughter, Aiyana's, turn. She was fifteen years old. I asked her to choose a place anywhere in the world and we would go there together for three weeks. With no hesitation, she firmly stated that she wanted to go to the Amazon jungle and meet the shaman about whom she had heard me tell many stories.

The jaguar shaman

I had already made a trip to South America in 1994 with a group of pharmacists and botanists who were all interested in setting up an ecological reserve that would be protected from the devastation going on in the rainforest. In addition, we were all eager to learn as much as possible about the healing properties of plants growing deep in the jungles. I was fortunate to be part of a walking tour of the Amazon Bushmaster Trail with Dr. Mark Plotkin, author of *Tales of a Shaman's Apprentice*. Despite the myriad of strange and peculiar insects and creatures that populated the dense undergrowth, I had observed that the native people walked freely through the jungle forest with little or no foot covering. It was a warm and humid spring day in November, so I brazenly decided on open sandals for the trek. Dr. Plotkin was speaking and identifying features of the local plants, while we all scribbled notes into our journals. The sensation of insects running over my toes was secondary to the information I wanted to glean on this trip. I was standing looking at a plant known as cat's claw, in its early stages, and I remember feeling the sting of an ant bite on my left foot. A few minutes later, I felt my throat tighten and my chest constrict, so I lingered behind the group. Then I realized I was going into anaphylactic shock. Two thoughts crossed my mind at that terrifying moment. The first was the realization that we were almost four hours from the nearest city and hospital, and theoretically I needed a hospital in six minutes. The second was that I was traveling with pharmacists; surely one of them had an epi-pen (epinephrine) or Benadryl or some form of antihistamine. But I couldn't get their attention as they were too far ahead of me by this time. What could I do? I felt myself going down for the count.

Suddenly I felt the strength of a man's body guiding me to lie down on a wooden platform. I looked up into the face of a Native Peruvian man who gazed back at me calmly and silently. He was short, stocky and typical of his people. He was holding a fresh plant in his hand and dipping it into a bucket of water. Again and again, he then shook the plant water over my body. At some point, there was smoke blowing into my face and all over my body and then he began singing a song in his own language. At this point, one of the South Americans from our group came back. He was able to translate.

As soon as my breath returned to normal, I asked him what was going on. Who was this man saving my life and what was the plant he carried? After a little cross dialogue between the translator and the shaman, the translator said, "Don Antonio was walking in the jungle and there was a ripple in the force and you were that ripple. His job was to straighten out the ripple." Immediately, I had visions of *Star Wars* and Luke Skywalker. "There is a ripple in the force, Luke!" To this day, I still wonder about the identity of the plant he used over me. And the smoke? Don Antonio eluded my questions, although I think I followed him around like a puppy dog for the next week. I wanted to learn more about his mysterious ways, and although he never confirmed for me the name of that plant, he shared many stories about the healing nature of the botanicals in his part of the world.

That was my first meeting with the shaman Don Antonio, known as the Jaguar Shaman. He is sympathetic to the spirit of the jaguar, or puma as it is known, which is native to the jungles of northeastern Peru.

Now, two years later, my daughter was curious enough to want to meet him, so we boarded the plane in Calgary, flew to Toronto, then onto Miami, and from there landed in Lima. After a four-hour wait in the Lima airport, we continued our trip by air to the deep Amazon jungle city of Iquitos. Still not able to rest, at Iquitos we hired a boat to make the four-hour journey down the Amazon River to a base camp. I still had no clue how I was going to actually find Don Antonio. After all, it wasn't like you could dial 1-800-SHAMAN, and get an update on his whereabouts in the jungle. He was known to spend time in the area of the base camp, but that was some two years back. My plan was that we would hire some local guides to see if they could find him. If that failed, I would stand on an ant hill until he came.

Finally, after almost thirty-two hours in transit, a bedraggled and travel-worn father and daughter saw the outline of the riverside base camp. The motor boat was small and we had sat huddled and exhausted staring into the murky Amazon waters, wondering quietly to ourselves about snakes and crocodiles and poisonous plants: the unknown. Our guide turned off the motor and we coasted silently toward the dock. We gathered up our bags and prepared to climb out of the boat. A Peruvian stood on the end of the dock. It was Don Antonio, the Jaguar Shaman. I almost fell out of the boat. There would be no search, because here he was, calmly and quietly greeting us after our long ordeal. He knew we were arriving, and had been pacing back and forth on the dock, as if waiting for our plane at an international airport.

For the next couple of weeks, Aiyana and I spent many days in the jungle with the shaman exploring the incredible beauty and mystery of Amazon insects and plants. Don Antonio was extremely open, telling me what the herbs were used for, and often even singing their songs for us. Of course, this was all through the services of a translator, as I cannot speak a bit of Yagua Indian, or Spanish, and he spoke no English and only a little Spanish, but we enjoyed ourselves nonetheless.

After a few days we went up to the Amazon Center for Environmental Education and Research, an ecological study area that was almost entirely in the canopy of the rainforest, some 115 feet above the ground. As we walked up the trail, I noticed a mushroom that I wanted to take a closer look at and check out. And yes, it was reishi *(Ganoderma lucidum)*, my favorite herb. In 1990, I had written a book on this herb, called *Reishi Mushroom: Herb of Spiritual Potency and Medical Wonder* and had been using it regularly in my clinic for the last decade or so. Here was wild reishi growing in the great shaman's territory. I was excited with my good fortune. The conversation protocol we had worked out over the last few days was that Don Antonio would point out plants to me, tell me their name, and maybe tell a story or two about its qualities. Sometimes he sang a song. Often, I would point out a plant and the same process would happen. So, I pointed to the reishi and asked about its medicinal properties. He answered that it had no medicinal properties. You can imagine the level of deflation and sadness I felt; my favorite healing herb and the great shaman was telling me in Peru there were no medicinal uses for it. I could not believe this.

The days lingered on and we saw many more exotic herbs, psychedelic colored frogs and all kinds of bizarre and interesting insects. One day, I was exploring for herbs and my daughter sat on a log with a beetle the size of a dinner plate on her leg. Affectionately, Don Antonio had brought her the prize beetle. Everything was going so well. Every day I was learning about several new herbs and soaking up the feeling you can get only deep in the Amazon jungle. A few days passed and I tried to slip the reishi mushroom in among a bunch of other plants we were examining. The same answer came back—there were no medicinal properties for the mushroom.

Before we knew it we only had one last day with Don Antonio before heading up to the Andes to hike the Inca trail to Machu Picchu. Determined, I decided to slip the mushroom into the conversation one more time, just in case. Well, I don't know if persistence paid off, whether I asked differently, or if the translator made the request differently, but I got a completely new story back this time.

Don Antonio said, "The plant you call reishi is not like the other plants we have looked at. It does not have medicinal properties like those. In fact, what you might think is the plant is really only the fruit, like a mango or lime. (This was truly amazing as Don Antonio had never been to school to study biology. Modern science knows that the fruiting body of a mushroom is connected to a large mycelium system, which is similar to the branching roots in a tree system.) He continued, "In fact the tree is underground and it is very, very large. It takes up many miles of the surrounding forest. It is also very, very old, being here before the jungles were. Because it has lived here a very long time, it is very wise; it knows all the plants and all the animals. So, when we have to go to the city and spend some time there, we often take this herb with us. It reminds us of the jungle. It can help us communicate with this underground tree back home and ground us in the Earth energy of the great jungle."

Once again, Don Antonio had amazed me. I had studied this plant for more than a decade and used it with many thousands of patients and he summed up in a few sentences what it really did. It grounded and connected you with the Earth energy. All the triterpenes, polysaccharides and other chemical units it contained did not really matter; nor did all the studies done in laboratories and clinics around the world. It came down to the simple statement that it helps tune us into Earth energy, Gaia. It helps us tune into the radio station R-E-I, S-H-I, the channel of Gaia, giving us a grounded feeling all day long.

Reishi and mental chatter

I was first introduced to reishi in the summer of 1986 by Dr. Wu, considered one of the world authorities in Fu Zheng (pronounced FOO-shen) an ancient and modern depiction of medicinal plants that work on the immune system. I was interviewing him in the famous Pu Chiang restaurant perched on top of the Hua Ting Shanghai Sheraton. He was studying herbs with adaptogenic properties, herbs that help a person adapt to a large range of physical, environmental, biological and personal stresses. After we talked about a number of herbs, Dr. Wu told me that the herb he felt was best was Ling Zhi (the Chinese name for reishi or *Ganoderma*). Dr. Wu impressed me so thoroughly with his knowledge of reishi that I began to use this herb extensively in my clinical practice and can say without reservation that it is the most important herb in the treatment of autoimmune or PNI issues. A common symptom of these issues is too much anxiety and mental chatter.

In China, they often use bylines to help the students remember the attributes of a medicinal plant. One of the bylines for Reishi is "to get rid of the knot in your chest." Reishi is also the major ingredient in a formula that has the byline, "to protect an academic from their own brain." These little "brain hook" memory aids, along with Don Antonio's statement of how it helps ground you into Earth (Gaia) energy, speak volumes for how it works.

Reishi is the best herb I have ever found to reduce brain chatter, repetitive thinking or circular arguments. For those cerebral types who live too much in their head, this herb is excellent. The "knot in the chest" can be interpreted to be constriction of the heart chakra. This can manifest as severe asthma, and reishi is a great asthmatic medicine. It also works on the heart and the circulation of the body, balancing both cholesterol and triglyceride levels.

Folklore

The reishi mushroom has been considered the most valuable herb of the Orient, outpacing even the reputation of ginseng. The mystical qualities attributed to this herb might be explained by the rarity of the plant: only two to three mushrooms are found for every 10,000 dead plum or hemlock logs, on which the mushroom grows. Sophisticated cultivation techniques now make reishi more available.

The nature of reishi mushroom is documented in *Shen Nung Tsao Ching*, where it is described as having the most extensive and effective healing powers. Since that time (56 BCE) it has been considered first amongst the higher herbs. Over the centuries it has gone by many names: happy herb, herb of spiritual potency, ten-thousand-year mushroom, miraculous chi, auspicious herb and good omen plant. Folklore has it that the herb was considered so valuable that if a person found one he or she would not even tell their closest friends or relatives.

In traditional Chinese medicine the list of traditional uses is long and includes nourishing, supplementing, toning, removing toxins and dispersing accumulation. It is indicated for neurasthenia, nervousness, dizziness, insomnia, high blood pressure, high cholesterol, chronic hepatitis, cancer, AIDS, nephritis, bronchial asthma, allergies, pneumonia, stomach disease, coronary heart disease, diabetes, angina, mushroom poisoning, fatigue and enhancing longevity. Reishi is often classed as an adaptogen (a substance that aids the body to resist a wide range of physical, biological and environmental stresses).

Studies on reishi

As we have seen, one of the biggest problems with autoimmune health issues is internal mental chatter. Reishi has been shown to reduce insomnia, anxiety, depression and paranoia. For respiratory-related problems, it demonstrated a 60 percent recovery rate in allergy-related chronic bronchitis, with improvement in 97.9 percent of the cases. Other studies have shown benefit for 87.5 percent of bronchial asthmatics with a cure rate of 48 percent. Reishi was shown to significantly inhibit histamine release and to be effective against Ig-E-related allergies.

Studies completed in Japan have confirmed that reishi can be responsible for arresting metastic cancer. The Japanese Cancer Society has found reishi effective against sarcomas.

It has been indicated for neurasthenia, nervousness, anxiety, dizziness, insomnia, high blood pressure, high cholesterol, chronic hepatitis, cancer, AIDS, nephritis, bronchial asthma, allergies, pneumonia, stomach disease, coronary heart disease, diabetes, syndrome X, angina, mushroom poisoning, fatigue, and for enhancing longevity.

Its antioxidant effect has been shown to be effective in scavenging hydroxyl radicals in blood plasma. For sinus problems, the cure rate is over 50 percent with approximately 80 percent effectiveness. Reishi protects from the effects of accumulated fatty acid and cholesterol, showing significant results in lowering blood lipids and fatty deposits in the liver. In studies on cholesterol and triglyceride levels, it significantly dropped their levels after two months.

Energetics

On an energetic level, it is listed as sweet and mild flavored with a warm property. Its action is nourishing, supplementing and tonifying. It removes toxins, disperses accumulation and stops tightness in the chest.

Reishi has never been studied for its effects on the subtle bodies, and is not available in essence form. However, its action does influence the emotional and/or mental body. It is used in powder or extract form.

Dosage

1–15 g daily, with 3–6 g being the most common recommendation.

St. Johns's wort *(Hypericum perforatum)*: the tranquil one

Depression often accompanies autoimmune disturbances, so I want to examine one of the best herbs for this symptom. How does St. John's wort, the much publicized herb for depression, really work? This question has been debated among academics and researchers in both Europe and North America for the last several years.

When I first started using St. John's wort in my clinic in the mid- to late-1980s, the herb was rarely used for depression because it was principally known as an antiviral. This was just after HIV was discovered as the cause of AIDS, and the natural medicine community was looking for a strong, natural antiviral. St. John's wort seemed to be one of the solutions, as not only did it function to destroy viruses but also was particularly effective for retroviruses. One of the chemicals in St. John's wort, hypericin, was shown to act as the antiviral agent.

However, the first major problem was the quantity required for therapeutic results—between 10 and 30 capsules a day to get the levels of hypericin needed. It seemed to control viruses for several of my AIDS patients. It was also beneficial for the growing new health issue, chronic Epstein-Barr virus, later renamed chronic fatigue syndrome (and subsequently determined not to be a virus, after all). The second problem was, of course, the expense and inconvenience of taking these large quantities of capsules. The third problem was more mysterious. Several of my patients, who went through the hassle and expense of swallowing these large quantities, found that they became "allergic" to commercial refrigeration units, complaining that refrigerators caused a full body sensation right down to their fingertips and toes, "like a dentist drilling into an unfrozen, sore tooth." This pain was acute and occurred only when they were within about 10 feet or so of a commercial refrigeration unit, like the kind found in a supermarket. Shopping was extremely unsettling for these people. Later, I learned that this was a known side effect of hypericin.

This side-effect captured my interest, because I suspected that there was some kind of electromagnetic interference going on in the etheric body between the St. John's wort and the electrical system of the refrigerator, which led me to believe that this herb worked more on the subtle bodies than the physical body. Not long after these strange events, herbal practitioners began to notice that St. John's wort seemed to alleviate depression for many people with dramatic health issues. Eventually, extensive research in Germany confirmed the antidepressant quality of the herb, which inspired a huge demand. Was the full-body tooth pain almost a homeopathic "proving" that was happening in these sensitive patients?

This remedy is used by homeopaths, in its diluted form, as the great remedy for injuries to nerves, especially in fingers, toes and nails. Excessive painfulness is a guiding symptom for its use as it relieves pain better than morphine. Its homeopathic mind attributes are anxiety, such as falling from heights, shock and melancholy. It is specific for puncture wounds, especially for pain after operations, when a person is cut by the scalpel. It is also used specifically for pain in the lower back, or the coccyx, after a fall on the tailbone or after childbirth.

Folklore

The history behind the name St. John's wort is in itself wonderful. This European native herb is called St. John's wort because it first flowers on St. John's Day, right before the summer solstice. Fortunately, it continues to flower all summer long, so there is ample time for harvesting the herb. The flowering at such an auspicious time was not lost on the medieval Catholic peasants. When viewed from the top, the small stems create a perfect cross. This symbolism became attached to the plant and the peasants came to believe that the plant offered protection for everything from lightning to witchcraft.

The scientific name *Hypericum perforatum* is also highly symbolic. The genus name comes from the Greek word *hypericon*, meaning to place "above the icon." This attribute was popularized in the Middle Ages, when the herb was considered to protect people against demons, witchcraft and lightning. If you hold the leaf up to the sunlight, you can see little perforations in it— hence the species name *perforatum*. This phenomena suggested its use for pin and needle perforations of the skin in the form of wounds. In turn, this fueled more belief that the plant could protect a person from occult voodoo practices (psychic attacks caused by poking pins into effigy dolls).

Paracelsus (1493–1541) considered it almost a universal medicine, again to purge the psychic energies of possession, ghosts and spooks. This applied to many forms of insanity and other health issues like epilepsy, schizophrenia, hallucinations and paralysis.

The famous German naturopath, Father Sebastian Kneipp, who created several water cures, said that this plant was the "perfume of God" and the "flower of the fairies." This is quite curious when you consider how revered the plant was to many American Indian tribes. Foreign to North America, the Europeans brought it over as a medicine, and by the 1800s it had completely naturalized to the local habitat. The question is, how did the Indian tribes learn of its medicinal value? Matthew Wood relates many great stories and insights about this herb in his excellent publication, *The Book of Herbal Wisdom*. He asked one of his teachers, an Indian elder, how the Native people knew so much about the use of this foreign plant. The story goes that the elder explained the European "little people" told the North American "little people" and they told their healers.

Wood claims that St. John's wort is a great remedy for the solar plexus, the center that is often associated with self-esteem issues. It also improves gut level instinct and, thus, will help deal with unconscious sensitivities.

Interestingly enough, this group of Indians used it to prevent witchcraft, saying that a witch cannot stand up when St. John's wort is present. Wood then goes on to illustrate this with some interesting case stories. He also relates how St. John's wort helps a person enter and leave dream states.

In Europe, St. John's wort was considered beneficial during children's stages of growth and for aging; for bed-wetting in young children; menstrual problems (cramping, irregularities and pain) and menopause. It is thought to be very useful for people with a sensitivity to weather changes (at the one-drop dosage level). I have used it extensively during winter months (at full dose) for seasonal affective disorder (SAD) with great success.

These interesting facts still do not answer the initial question: how does St. John's wort work? There is no doubt it alleviates mood disorders, as we use it for thousands of patients who come through the clinic every year, and it is more effective than most pharmaceutical antidepressants. One thing we do know is that it blossoms and matures when the sun is at its height in June each summer. In fact, levels of several of the active constituents are directly determined by the amount of available sunlight. In cloudy years, the chemical levels are low; in sunny years, higher. St. John's wort appears to concentrate sunlight. In fact, one of the risks with this herb is that if white-faced cows or sheep eat large quantities, they develop sun sensitivity and grow huge skin ulcers. This observation lead to the erroneous idea that people should not go out in the sun when using the herb therapeutically. In an Internet poll I was involved in, only six documented cases of this side effect were reported. The poll consisted of feedback from more than 100 million combined doses per year from both practitioners and manufacturers. So, there is a 0.006 percent chance that this might happen, far below the level of any real risk.

However, this function of St. John's wort gives us a clue as to how it works. Depression can be likened to a dark cloud overshadowing a person's life. St. John's wort appears to bring a ray of sunshine into cloudy situations. I think of it as a herbal solar battery, which is why I continue to give it to SAD people.

Studies on St. John's wort

From a clinical standpoint, we know that the alkaloid has a tonic effect on the ventricles of the heart, the aorta and arterioles, and is also useful for pulmonary complaints, bladder trouble, suppression of urine, dysentery, worms and nervous depression.

Even small amounts have been found effective for increasing blood flow to stressed tissue, especially punctures. This blood flow has also shown to be hypotensive, reducing capillary fragility and enhancing uterine tone.

St. John's wort has antibacterial and antiviral activity against a range of organisms including tuberculosis, Gram positive organisms, *Micrococcus, Bacillus* and influenza A/PR8. Tests at the U.S. National Cancer Institute have found an extract of St. John's wort shows promise against cancer.

Subtle effects

From a flower essence perspective, St. John's wort illuminates consciousness and gives light-filled awareness and strength. It is used for people who are experiencing overly expanded states that may lead to psychic and physical vulnerability; for deep fear and disturbed dreams. I find it useful, in general, for people who are emotionally oversensitive or overly receptive. It is recommended for people who have an overly active psychic life—the astral body expands greatly during sleep, and this expansiveness can be associated with attacks from elemental or other entities, especially during sleep. Again, we find this theme of protection from psychic attack has stayed with the plant throughout the ages.

Dosage

- Physical
Capsule	300 mg, 3 times daily
Infusion	1–2 tablespoons
Fluid extract (1:1)	20–30 drops; 3 times daily

- Etheric
    Fresh fluid extract   1–3 drops; 1–3 times daily
- Astral (emotional)
    Flower essence   5 drops; 3 times daily or as needed
- Mental
    Homeopathic   6x–30x; 3 times daily or as needed

Kava kava (*Piper methysticum*): the relaxed mediator

Sitting under a palm tree, in the cool breeze off the ocean, a circle of virgin village girls in the South Pacific chew the dried roots of the revered kava kava plant. They spit the macerated root, mixed with saliva, onto a leaf. This is mixed with cold water. A coconut-full is given to each of the village elders to drink. These mildly euphoric drinks help the elders communicate clearly with each other and even the gods, due to the calm meditative state that it delivers. This scene has been playing itself out over and over throughout the centuries in the South Pacific.

Maybe we could all learn something from these wise elders today. Kava's use as a ceremonial herb could also be adapted for many arbitration situations. It provides a simple way to calm down the participants so they contribute positively to the communication, instead of responding from a place of emotional anger.

Long ago, on some of the Polynesian Islands, young men would get restless and want to go kick up a ruckus on other local islands. They would get together and form a war party, just like many other tribal societies did at that time around the world. They would get themselves all riled up and launch an attack. When they approached the next island, hopefully an elder would be present to try to develop a diplomatic solution to the events, but his young bucks would be more interested in fighting the attacking "wimps."

The elder would bring out some of the strong "war kava" and they would all drink it as part of the ceremony, similar to the way the Northern Plains Indians, where I come from, would pass around the peace pipe. After they drank this strong drink, the participants would start to calm down. Then after a while the warriors would say, "You know if we fight, some of us are bound to get hurt. We'll lose blood and maybe even a limb, possibly be laid up for weeks. You know, another drink of that kava you have sure would be good."

You see, it's hard to fight when you consume kava. In fact, I have often used it as part of family counseling in the clinic. After taking kava, it is hard to act from that emotional place where anger lives. Calmness is only one of its first lessons. If you can learn to listen, kava will teach you more.

Is there any truth to the stories that kava kava can calm you both mentally and physically? Modern scientific research bears out the validity of these ancient myths and practices.

Folklore

Kava kava (*Piper methysticum*) has been used in the South Pacific for its euphoric calming effect, but it has also been employed to relax muscles, for muscle aches and to treat epilepsy, toothaches, sore throats, gout, rheumatism, bronchitis, menstrual cramps and menopausal problems as well as some sexually transmitted diseases. In modern-day South Pacific, there are local bars, called talking bars, which serve kava drinks for the after-work crowd, much as Americans relax with an after-work cocktail. The consumer drinks the kava, relaxes and chats with others in the bar, washing away the day-to-day stresses. Kava has the added benefit of not being addictive or abusive to the liver, like alcohol. The European community and the U.S. show a steady increase in the use of this herb over the last several years. Many new kava products continue to appear in the marketplace.

How does this herb work? There are six major active ingredients (kavalactones) in kava. Even though there have been many attempts to synthesize a pharmaceutical drug from the derivatives, it has been shown that the herb's activity depends on a blend of all six to achieve its potency. Nature triumphs again, as there are no synthetic pharmaceutical analogs ready for market in the near future. The ratio between the specific chemicals will produce different effects. The kavalactones have been compared by many to tranquilizers such as Valium in their effect. Unlike synthetic tranquilizers, kava enhances the ability to communicate, sharpens the senses and leaves the individual with an alert mind. I have used kava kava, in combination with other herbs, in my clinical practice for more than twenty years. We employ it mostly as a muscle relaxant; it eases chiropractic adjustments, while helping them hold longer. We also use it for professional athletes. By mildly relaxing the muscles, kava increases the flexibility, while enhancing mental clarity, and seems to increase an athlete's winning potential.

In addition, we use it for many cases of cystitis or bladder infections, as it contributes to the reduction of bladder infection in three ways. One, it has a strong antimicrobial effect in the body, which can reduce the infection in the bladder. Two, the kavalactones have a numbing effect in the mouth when taken as a tea. These same constituents have a numbing effect on the bladder, soothing the pain in that area, even when taken in a capsule form.

Three, many people get bladder inflammation from slight spasms in the bladder and associated tubes; kava helps reduce these spasms.

Studies on kava

There have been more than 800 scientific references listed in the large body of literature on this herb. Here are a few recent highlights of the research on this South Pacific pepper plant. The kavalactones have their action mainly on the reticular formation of the brain stem, which creates a relaxing effect on the muscles, digestive and urinary tract. In addition, kava has been shown to:

- Increase recognition of new words and concepts related to the memory of older words and concepts. This would point to its ability to improve communication and aid in resolving conflict.
- Have a neuroprotective activity in the brain, which has the potential to reduce the damage related to strokes.
- Relax the limbic (emotional) centers in the brain by reducing anxiety, assisting sleep and calming emotional problems related to menopause.
- Produce a pain-relieving effect.
- Reduce the affects of amphetamines.

One randomized, double-blind, placebo-controlled study shows how daily stress and nonclinical levels of anxiety in adults can be reduced by the use of kava in formula, in as little as two weeks. Subjects using kava for four weeks all had reduced symptoms on eight measures of stress.

If muscles are tight, or lack of flexibility limits a fitness program, kava is worth a closer look. Fibromyalgia patients often find using kava as a nutritional supplement helps to reduce the muscle aches and pains so characteristic of this disorder.

CHAPTER SEVEN ☆ Herbs as Teachers

Will we see the day when the mediator's office gives a round of kava extract before participants work through business or domestic disputes? The future holds many possibilities for this master herb.

Energetics

In his book *Planetary Herbology* Dr. Michael Tierra lists kava kava as pungent, bitter and warm, and entering the liver and kidney meridians. Dr. A. A. Culbreth, a nineteenth-century Eclectic medical doctor and professor, wrote in his *materia medica* that the odor was faint, characteristic, taste aromatic, pungent, bitter— more or less anesthetic.

Homeopathically, Boericke (a famous 1920s homeopath) said kava was used for a person who is silent and drowsy, who has an intolerance to dreams and loss of muscular power. It is used for highly sensitive people, who have an exhausted minds and constantly need to change position—which can temporarily reduce pain by diverting attention. Kava kava is also used to increase urination, especially for cystitis.

Toxicity

There has been much controversy about kava and liver toxicity since 2001, when both Germany and Switzerland reported several cases of liver problems potentially related to kava consumption. An independent study was conducted by Professor Waller, a respected epidemiologist from the University of Chicago. The findings from this study showed no relationship between the liver problems of these patients and their consumption of kava.

Dosage

Crude herb	1–2 grams daily
Fluid extract	60 drops
Homeopathic	single drop and low potency

Skullcap *(Scutellaria lateriflora)*: the psychic soother

The gentle soothing effect of skullcap is profound and most suitable for the anxiety that accompanies many autoimmune conditions. For a long time now there has been intense debate about whether or not skullcap really has any therapeutic action. I, along with thousands of patients, can certainly attest that it works quite well, especially for those who also have autoimmune-related problems. The debate appears to come from two distinct factors: one, its effects are certainly subtle and, two, results depend on whether it is prepared fresh or dried.

The action of skullcap is gentle, as it calms down excessive mental processing. If you use it for other types of nervousness, it might not work as well—simply because it is the wrong herb for the situation. The writings of the Eclectics (1800–1940), prominent school medical doctors using botanical remedies, show they also debated whether it should be a fresh tincture or a dried tincture. Most of them found it worked best as a fresh tincture. Since we grow this herb on our farm, I have been able to observe the action in both forms. Although I do feel the fresh tincture has a stronger action, the dry nevertheless gives results. I almost always use the fresh tincture now, if available, and it usually is. I have also found the dried herb useful as an infusion tea, especially for teething babies.

Skullcap (like reishi) has a direct action on excessive circular or repetitive thinking (what nineteenth-century doctors called monomania), and is also beneficial for nervousness and mental and physical exhaustion. In the late 1800s and early 1900s, the Eclectics described a health issue called neurasthenia, which appears in their definition to be the same disease as chronic fatigue syndrome and fibromyalgia. Skullcap was considered specific for neurasthenia. Skullcap is also effective for releasing the type of muscle tension found in fibromyalgia. Functional heart problems related to nervousness, such as heart palpitations, can be treated very effectively with this herb.

Folklore

Folklore has it that skullcap's major influence is on the central and sympathetic nervous systems. It has been used for hydrophobia (rabies, thus one of its names is "mad dog" skullcap), St. Vitus' Dance, neuralgia, insomnia, excitability, restlessness, rickets, headaches, hiccups, incessant coughing, hypertension, snake bites, to promote menstruation and for poisonous bites. It was noted in James' *Herbal* as early as 1743. The Cherokee and Iroquois used skullcap to induce vomiting, and for a variety of problems including gynecological ailments, as an abortifacient and as an antidiarrheal.

Studies on skullcap

The calming effect of skullcap has been attributed to a major constituent, scutellarin, and has been used to treat hiccups, insomnia and nervous disorders. A 70 percent methanol extract of the whole root of this species with flavonoids present showed antiarthritic and anti-inflammatory action. Chinese scullcap (*S. baicalensis*) root has shown significant antiallergenic and anti-inflammatory properties.

Skullcap has shown an antihistamine effect, as well as inhibiting contraction of the vas deferens. Heart rate has been shown to be reduced. These studies indicate its physiological calming action.

Therapeutic Action

Antispasmodic, nervine, tonic, antipyretic, anaphrodisiac and a slight astringent.

Energetics

In Chinese medicine, scullcap (herbage of a related species *S. barbata*) is pungent with a neutral property. It cleanses heat, removes toxins, disperses stagnancy and controls bleeding and pain. The root of *S. baicalensis* is bitter and cold, entering the heart, lung, gall bladder, small intestine and colon meridians. The action is to quell fire and clear heat, especially in the upper burner, drain damp heat, and calm the fetus, preventing spontaneous miscarriages.

In his book *The Energetic of Western Herbs* Colorado herbalist Holmes lists skullcap as bitter, a bit astringent, cold and dry, having secondary qualities of relaxing, restoring and stimulating while stabilizing movement. It enters the heart and kidney meridians while influencing the heart, kidney, urogenital organs, autonomic and central nervous system, brain and spine. The organism is air. Tierra lists skullcap as bitter and cool, and able to influence the heart and liver meridian.

Homeopathically, Boericke lists scutellaria as a nervous sedative where nervous fear predominates and cardiac irritability is present. He suggests it is specified for infants to reduce nervousness and spasms during teething, and for nervous weakness after influenza in adults. The associated mental attributes for homeopathic usage are fear of some calamity, inability to fix attention and confusion, restless sleep and frightful dreams, and migraine, worse over right eye.

Dosage

Powder	15–30 grains
Infusion	3 oz
Tincture	10–40 drops
Fluid extract	1/4 tsp
Homeopathic	1 drop level to 30x potency

Siberian ginseng (*Eleuthrococcus senticosus*): the calming energizer

I consider Siberian ginseng to be the tai chi master of all the herbs; it gives strength and energy while at the same time producing a calming effect. People with many of the stress-related health issues we have mentioned need a tonic. However, most tonics backfire by making the person more wired and increasing insomnia. Not Siberian ginseng. In our clinic, we recommend this remedy most often for athletic energy, chronic fatigue, fibromyalgia, when a person is under too much stress, recovering from an illness (convalescence) and for a wide variety of calming functions.

Folklore

This plant was used as a folk remedy for heart ailments, insomnia, hemiplegia, hypertension and rheumatism. It has also been employed to restore vigor, memory, good appetite and longevity. In China, it is used to lower cholesterol, cure impotence and increase blood oxygen.

Studies on Siberian Ginseng

There is a wealth of scientific data supporting the use of Siberian ginseng to improve health. Many of the studies emphasize the herb's usefulness for the immune system in withstanding exposure to stress. It has been shown to have immunostimulating activity, with increased immune activities shown in both test tubes and humans. One dramatic study demonstrated that children with bacterial intestinal infections recovered faster when given Siberian ginseng extract along with antibiotics in contrast to antibiotics alone. This was accompanied by an increase in many immune mediated cells. It is considered that these actions function by influence in the pituitary-adrenocortical system, similar to Asian ginseng. Much of this seems to be due to both the tonic and calming effect it has on the user.

The extract of Siberian ginseng increases physical performance, growth, survival rate and protein metabolism in organ and muscle tissue. The extract can increase a person's resistance to heat exposure and double the survival time during chronic irradiation. In females, the activation rate of steroidal receptors was higher in the uterus (including response to estrogen) when it was ingested. Used along with chemotherapy, it has been shown to reduce side effects of radiation treatment. It has also been shown to reduce blood sugar.

Other areas in which studies confirm positive effects from Siberian ginseng extract are immune system of cancer patients; heart structure in myocardial infarctions, arrhythmias and other heart diseases; diabetes; antimicrobial action and prenatal prevention of congenital developmental anomalies. It has also been shown to produce anti-edemic, diuretic, antihypertensive and anti-inflammatory effects.

Therapeutic Action

Adaptogen (increases resistance to physical, biological, environmental and personal stresses).

Energetics

Tierra describes Siberian ginseng as acrid, sweet and bitter; influencing the liver and kidney acupuncture meridians.

Dosage

Powder	3–15 g daily
Tincture	10–50 drops daily

Red root *(Ceanothus americanus)*: the enlivening muse

The medicinal part of this herb is the root, which is covered in tiny nodules, suggesting that it might be helpful for the lymphatic system. A toxic lymphatic system or, in traditional Chinese medicine terms, stagnation of the spleen, is characteristic of those diagnosed with CFS, FM and similar categories. A cross section of the root is red, suggesting it works on blood. Allopathic doctors used it to stop hemorrhaging during operations in the mid-1800s, but its major use, by allopaths, herbalists and homeopaths alike, was for glands, the lymphatic system and specifically as a spleen remedy.

The old herbals, from the turn of the century in America, describe many uses for this plant: a remedy for swollen glands, lymphatic stagnation, edema, pelvic congestion, enlargement and inflammation of the spleen, violent shortness of breath (caused by a swollen spleen), chronic bronchitis with profuse mucus, and pain in the liver or back. Less popular uses included loss of appetite, excess weight loss, general weakness, pain and weakness in the umbilical region, anemia, pallor, diarrhea, bearing down pain in the abdomen and rectum, constant urging to urinate and profuse menstruation. There are also accounts of its use for swollen sore throat, swollen prostrate and breast problems. Red root was listed as most effective for symptoms that are worse in damp, cold weather.

Even though this is an extensive list, stagnation of the spleen (lymphatic system) is the key here. Michael Moore, often considered the godfather of American herbalism, describes in his book *Medicinal Plants of the Desert and Canyon* an interesting experiment. He mixed some of his blood with the juice of this plant and observed it under a dark field microscope. He showed that a small electrical charge occurred that separated the red blood cells from the blood protein on the microscope slide. He then theorized from this data that the red root forced the red blood cells and proteins into the center of the capillaries, thus leaving the walls free for the interstitial fluid (lymphatic) to penetrate the walls. He interpreted this action to mean that red root will help the blood deliver both lymph and nutrients to the tissue more effectively—which Moore believes is behind the traditional concept of reducing lymphatic stagnation.

Energetics

Similarly, Matthew Wood describes red root in association with the spleen and the emotion melancholia, which he expands to include excessive thoughts, brooding and introspection, all emotions related to the health issues we are examining. This line of interpretation is found throughout the writings of several homeopaths and herbalists. Clearly, today we would term this condition simply as depression. Melancholy is also associated with lack of direction, purpose or creativity, or being in an artistic funk.

Mimi Kamp, a herbalist from the southwestern United States, recommends that red root be used by "people who show the inability to think themselves out of a problem." In other words, it helps a person reduce circular arguments, which produce no resolution. As Wood points out, the psychological faculty most closely associated with the spleen is imagination. Both the Chinese and the ancient Greeks stated that the spleen was associated with the Earth and a strong sense of being grounded. As we have repeatedly found at the clinic, emotionally sensitive individuals who maintain excessively busy lives, without allowing time for relaxation and reflection, risk severing all connection with the imaginative and creative aspects of life. Eventually, this takes its toll on health.

Dosage

We strongly recommend not exceeding suggested dosage without seeking the advice of a practitioner who understands the use of this herb. Some people do experience toxic reactions, indicated by a swollen tongue, with as little as 10 drops. Large continuous doses, more than 20 drops, can produce sticking pain in the spleen, increased by motion, inability to lie on left side and enlargement of the spleen in healthy individuals. These same symptoms may occur in the liver, with enlargement and congestive pain worse on touch, and general weakness.

Tincture	1–3 drops; 1–4 times daily
Homeopathic	3x to 3C

Barberry *(Berberis vulgaris)*: the protector

The primary symptom guiding the use of barberry is the feeling of being invaded. One of my long-term patients gave birth to extremely premature twins who both survived, one 1.7 pounds and the other 2.9 pounds. The smallest (Sammie, a boy) had to live his first eight months connected to life-support equipment.

For the first six months after coming off life support Sammie made good progress, and then everything stopped. For more than a month he gained no weight and seemed to be suffering from malnutrition. Barberry came to mind, as this little child had spent the first part of his life in a completely invaded space, hooked up to multiple tubes of life support and subjected to continuous probing for various tests. He was given 1 drop of barberry twice daily for a month and he started to gain weight; some seven years later, Sammie is a very happy and healthy boy.

Barberry is traditionally given to fight off microorganisms, and is also an excellent tonic, especially for delicate and weak children. I also find it useful for patients who need protection, especially in the gastrointestinal tract. About four years ago, Wendy (twenty-two years old) came in with what sounded like horrible news. While traveling in the tropics she had picked up some parasites. She went to her doctor who, after the examination, said that her digestive tract was full of eggs that were about to hatch in about 1–2 weeks and that once hatched would likely eat right through the lining of her bowel. She could expect to die in about three weeks. Again, barberry tincture was brought in, this time at 20 drops three times daily, which helped protect her digestive tract while some antiparasitic herbs were employed successfully. Today, she is in good shape and several tests have shown no return of the parasites.

Folklore

Barberry has traditionally been used as an excellent remedy for digestive and liver problems. It is also suggested for jaundice.

Barberry has been used since the time of the ancients. Barberry is a famous Indian remedy and one of the most valuable herbs, and is unequalled for normalizing liver secretions. It is an excellent tonic for the delicate and weak (especially children) and alleviates anemia and general malnutrition in just a few weeks. It regulates the digestive system, lessens the size of the spleen and removes obstructions in the intestinal tract.

The Blackfoot Indians called barberry *oti-to-gue* and used the steeped, peeled, dried root to check rectal hemorrhages, dysentery and stomach troubles. The bark of the root contains an alkaloid (berberine) that promotes bile secretion. When cayenne is used as a "carrier" and matched with barberry, the resulting formula will exhibit superior stimulatory effects on the liver. The alkaloids in the root also tend to dilate the blood vessels and thereby lower blood pressure.

A tincture of the root is helpful in urinary complaints, especially herpes simplex. The Blackfoot Indians would apply either fresh berries or an infusion of the root to open boils. The berries were also used for kidney troubles. Externally, the infused root was applied to wounds as an antiseptic. The root was also chewed and then applied for the same purpose. As horse medicine, the berries were soaked in water and the resulting juice was given to a coughing horse. Human body sores were also treated with the infusion of the root. Barberry was listed in John Gerard's seventeenth-century book, *The Herbal,* and for centuries was used in Mongolia, Russia and Europe for gall-bladder problems, hemorrhage and inflammation. The Navaho, Paiute and Shoshone were the most notable of a handful of tribes who used a number of *Berberis* species in North America. The plant was used for a broad range of ailments and was also included in certain ceremonies.

Studies on Barberry

As an immunostimulatory substance, the active constituent (berberine) has been shown to increase the blood supply to the spleen, while increasing the activity of immune system cells (macrophages). It has shown activity against tumor systems.

Barberry's antibiotic effect is quite astounding, inhibiting organisms at much lower concentration than most antibiotics. Barberry is effective against a large array of microorganisms, increasing in activity with pH levels. It is a stimulant on the myocardium in low doses; depressant in high doses. Barberry is a mild anesthetic for the mucous membranes. It reduces fever better than aspirin. Barberry is also known to be anticonvulsant, sedative, hypotensive, uterotonic and cholerectic.

Therapeutic Action

Barberry is a bitter tonic, stomachic, alterative and mild purgative that regulates digestion and is useful in treating diarrhea.

Energetics

In traditional Chinese medicine, a related species, *B. sargentianae,* has a bitter flavor with cold property.

Holmes says barberry is bitter and astringent, being cold and dry, with secondary qualities of astringing, decongesting, relaxing and restoring, while having a sinking movement. Barberry enters the spleen, stomach, liver and gall bladder meridians, acting on the liver, gall bladder, spleen, intestine and blood with an organism of warmth.

Dosage

Average dose	2.0 g
Decoction or infusion	15–60 ml (1:20 bark in H_2O)
Homeopathic mother tincture as drops up to 30x	

CHAPTER EIGHT

Body-Mind
Therapies

❖

My most challenging patients have taught me the importance of having more than herbs at my disposal; they have also shown me—as has the current research—that in addition to the stress-related symptoms so typical of autoimmune disorders, we often find similar emotional patterns. We have explained how herbs, in flower essence or homeopathic forms, can be used as a treatment for the emotional body. This chapter explores other kinds of therapies, some of which we employ in the clinic, that assist the process of emotional clearing and balancing. Remember, all these therapies are used to improve health by increasing a harmonious flow of communication between the physical body and the subtle bodies, thereby reducing autoimmune attacks. Here are five specific treatment areas:

- Somatic work to release the physical body trauma
- Oral dose items, such as herbs, flower essences and homeopathic remedies
- Creativity without perfectionism
- Energy psychology to aid in releasing emotional miasms or blocks
- Creative visualization exercises to help give you a firm direction for focus

Somatic work

The area of somatic (muscle release) work has a broad range of practical and beneficial applications that we will divide into two categories: passive and active. Examples of passive somatic work are various forms of body work, such as some types of massage, Rolfing, osteopathy, specific forms of chiropractic, craniosacral therapy, myofascial release, acupuncture, acupressure and shiatsu. A number of the more common forms of active somatic release include tai chi, yoga, creative movement, walking meditation, Pilates, Feldenkrais exercises and Alexander technique. There is no sharp line of demarcation between these therapies—some body-work has both active and passive components. As we will see, some forms of creative release, such as drumming, contain the attributes of active somatic release. The benefits of somatic release methods have been explained by focusing on two principal mechanisms, the structural integrity and vibratory energetic of the body.

There is no doubt that one of the strongest entraining forces for us, on the physical level, is the Earth's gravitational force, which affects our every activity and all parts of the physical body. The importance of alignment and posture on a daily basis was first investigated by the surgeon Joel Goldthwait and his colleagues at Harvard Medical School in the early twentieth century. They studied how many of our physiological processes, in order to work efficiently, rely on the proper alignment with gravity. Ida Rolf (herself a physicist) expanded on Goldthwaite's work to show that many emotions are functionally involved with the body's structural integrity and its relationship to gravity.

Alignment and structure in the physical body have been likened to a tensegrity, which underlies the principle of geodesic domes, tents, sailing vessels and many other stick-and-wire models. A tensegrity system is characterized by a continuous tensional net-work (tendons) connected by a discontinuous set of compressive elements (bones or struts) (see Figure 8.1). The structure forms a stable yet dynamic system that interacts efficiently and resiliently with forces acting upon it.

The spine is like a tensegrity mast. The various ligaments form "slings" that are capable of supporting the weight of the body without applying compression forces to the vertebra and intervertebral disc. Imbalance in one part of the body will cause the rest of the body to compensate for the fluctuation, thereby creating further imbalance throughout the system. For example, if one set of ligaments in the vertebrae is too tight or too loose it will throw off the spine's structure, and will inevitably affect the internal organs.

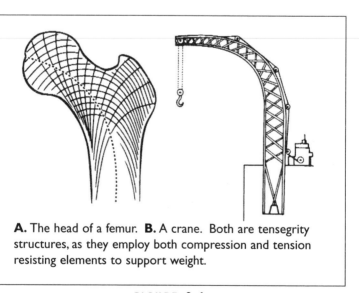

A. The head of a femur. **B.** A crane. Both are tensegrity structures, as they employ both compression and tension resisting elements to support weight.

FIGURE **8.1**

Sitting at a computer with shoulders tensed and the spine curved, or standing with the body's weight unevenly distributed and favoring one hip, are examples of common habits that affect the structural integrity of the entire body. These effects are partially due to the flexibility of the living tensegrity—a continuous semiconductor vibratory network—thereby allowing the body worker's energy to directly influence the entire living matrix, down to the cellular level. This ripple effect is one of the ways that Qi Chong, Rolfing, therapeutic touch and many other modalities work.

Since this tensegrity network is both a structural and vibratory continuum, any restriction due to poor postural alignment and structural problems will affect the energetic negatively throughout the body. The opposite is equally true. Improving the structure and alignment of the spine keeps the network in focus with gravity, and improves the energetic quality of the body. As explained in earlier chapters, this ligament structure can function down to the level of integrins (the "glue" for every cell) and influence the cytoskeleton at the cellular level. Recent scientific research has shown that a breakdown at the integrins level plays a key role in arthritis, heart disease, stroke, osteoporosis and the spread of cancer.

This approach is comprehensively defined in J. L. Oschman's book *Energy Medicine: The Scientific Basis,* wherein he shows how both toxins and electrical charges can get trapped in tissue and cause functional problems, both physically and emotionally. By releasing these "tensions" we become more physically functional and do not have to suffer from all the signs of aging. In our culture, there is a widely held misconception that these accumulated imbalances and discomforts are associated purely with aging and cannot be reversed. Many types of body therapies have proved the opposite. Developing body awareness to improve alignment, posture and free movement reduces the negative impacts of age and gravity.

Emotional issues stored in the subtle astral or etheric body can create negative changes in the various muscular structures of the body. Conversely, physical trauma can take its toll emotionally and cause blockages in the chakras or subtle bodies. It is a two-way street. As already explained, it is necessary to determine the center of gravity of the health issue: is it more physical or more emotional? Our physical body needs structural and postural integrity for healing to happen. This is the basic theory behind Rolfing, which by getting the physical body back in alignment with gravity not only assists physical performance but also improves emotional health. At the risk of repeating myself: If any area is restricted or constricted, you will have a more difficult time feeling the emotions associated with that area.

For example, the person who shows a concave alignment of the spine in the region of the upper back and chest is often attempting to protect the heart region. This frequently seen hollowed-out posture suggests a need to protect the self from pain and the heart from exposure. The opposite movement pattern, with the arms thrown wide open and the chest lifted, exposes the heart—a posture we associate with joy. Each postural pattern and habit has an associated emotional state. The body never lies.

Not only does passive therapy help body workers to realign the tensegrity network; many of the active somatic or movement-based release techniques will achieve similar results. This of course includes ancient systems like yoga, tai chi and various forms of Qi Chong, as well as contemporary forms such as Alexander technique and Body-Mind Centering. Free movement is essential for health. All of these movement therapies help the physical body better communicate within itself and with the subtle bodies. By communication, we refer to the flow of body fluids, the flow of neural impulses, the free movement of joints and the flow of electromagnetic vibration through the semi-conducting tensegrous living matrix. This will inevitably improve the flow via the acupuncture meridians and the chakra system.

I have found that both chronic fatigue syndrome and fibromyalgia patients benefit considerably by adopting some of form of somatic body work into their schedule. If any part of the hologram is upset, it will reflect in all parts of the hologram. In other words, specific emotional blocks will show up in the physical body or, conversely, signs in the physical body will help us interpret emotional issues that might be clouding the flow of energy in our subtle bodies. Many of my patients, especially those with fibromyalgia, have very precise aches in specific muscles.

Louise Hay and emotional patterns in the body

I see specific emotional patterns and temperaments in many of my patients with the same autoimmune-related concerns. This seems to mesh well with what Beth Hedva, Peter Levine and Stuart Heller are saying: that emotions can become frozen into the body. In Louise Hay's little book, *Heal Your Body,* she helps interpret patterns of emotional trauma in the body, and her book *You Can Heal Your Life* is constructive and helpful. Her books are a gold mine of information to help interpret how somatic issues relate to emotional problems. I had really come to respect her work after I found several of my immune-compromised patients, especially AIDS patients, a few of whom ceased to be HIV positive, go through her programs and make miraculous turnarounds.

Louise Hay relates various parts of the body to emotional issues. For example, if a person has a problem in his or her hand, we see the hand as a metaphor or association with a specific feeling; he or she might have a feeling of letting things slip through the fingers or possibly hold onto something too tight. I would not want to say that these associations are always accurate; however, they provide good general directions to help pinpoint which areas to look at. My clinical estimate is that they lead one in the right direction about 75 percent of the time. Here is a broad overview of Louise Hay's associations (more details can be found in her books):

Hair—feeling of strength; tension contributes to a strangling of the hair follicles, so they cannot grow properly.

Ears—something we do not want to hear.

Eyes—something we do not want to see.

Headaches—come for invalidation of self or sense of having done something that makes the individual feel wrong.

Sinus—represents being irritated by someone in your life, someone close to you.

Neck and throat—the ability to be flexible in our thinking. Being able to see the other side of a question or another person's point of view. Problems in the neck often come from being stubborn.

Throat—ability to "speak up" for ourselves. We do not feel we have the right or are unable to stand up for ourselves.

Arms—the ability and capacity to embrace the experiences of life.

Hands—we feel we are letting things slip through our fingers; or we hold onto something too long.

Fingers—show where we need to relax and let go. Thumbs represent mental worry. The index finger is anger and fear involving ego. The middle finger has to do with sex and anger (giving someone the finger). The ring finger represents both union and grief. The little finger has to do with family and pretending.

Back—our support system: problems with our backs mean we usually do not feel supported. The upper back has to do with emotional support, the middle back with guilt and the lower back with feeling "burnt out" either emotionally or financially.

Lungs—relate to taking and giving ; in other words, we cannot take life in or feel we do not have the right to live life to its fullest. Emphysema and heavy smoking are ways of denying or hiding from life (smoke screen).

Breast—our mothering aspect and can indicate either "over-mothering" or a feeling of inadequacy in our ability to mother.

Heart—the seat of love, with blood representing joy. If we deny love and joy in our lives, our blood gets sluggish and our heart becomes damaged.

Stomach—the digestion of new ideas and experiences. Often when a person is afraid to assimilate new experiences, stomach problems arise.

Genitals—represent either our most feminine or most masculine part. When we do not feel comfortable about our sexuality or feel dirty and sinful, we can manifest problems in this area.

This information is useful but many of my patients had very precise aches in specific muscles. This was particularly true for fibromyalgia patients. Since Louise Hay doesn't classify specific muscle pain in terms of emotions, I searched for material and found some insights in the field of bodynamic somatic developmental psychology. In particular, there was a book containing a group of articles edited by Ian MacNaughton called *Embodying the Mind & Minding the Body*. Besides several interesting discussions on somatic pain and their relationship to specific emotional issues, it has a list of muscles and the corresponding emotions. I started applying this information to my fibromyalgia patients and others with muscle pain, and found it helped me follow the right direction of inquiry and treatment. One of the articles by Bandelli's Laokoon and Babinetto Uffizi, Firenze, and embraced by the Society of Body-namic Somatic Developmental Psychology, lists some of the muscles and their associated emotions (see www.mind-bodyharmony.com for positions of the muscles and muscle groups):

Face muscles—receiving impressions and social/emotional signaling, expressing feelings, social space and dominance.

Eye and ear muscles—the ability to focus and orientate to short- and long-term planning.

Jaw, mouth and tongue muscles—vocal expression and the ability to incorporate and expel emotional or physical nourishment and respond to tastes and "digestibility".

Throat muscles—vocal expression, talking; balancing the head with the body; thoughts and feelings.

Neck muscles—hold the head up and represent "keeping one's head"; orientation, willpower and pride.

Shoulder elevators—carry emotional burdens and aid in keeping one's balance when on unsure mental/emotional footing.

Shoulder dorsal adductors and rotators—connect the core self and action; the ability to receive support from others and self-protection; creating personal space.

Shoulder joint (extensors, flexors, ab- [away from] and ad- [toward] ductors)—range in interpersonal activities and personal space; reaching out, touching, pushing and holding on to self-worth.

Elbow flexor muscle—pulling toward and holding on.

Elbow extensors—pushing away, throwing, holding at a distance.

Forearm rotators—giving and receiving, closing and opening to exchanges.

Wrist flexors, extensions, radial and ulnar [arm] flexors—fine control and positioning of social and interpersonal actions; modification of behavior to suit present company.

Finger flexors (abductors and adductors)—touching, holding and investigating of larger and fine adjustments in perception and handling; the basis of cognitive grasp and the ability to absorb and emit.

Finger extensors—letting go, reaching out and making fine adjustments in boundaries.

Thumb and little finger opposers—synthesis and refined focus, sensitivity to minute expression, reading and writing skills.

Pectorals and serratus anterior—superficial contact, self-worth and power of intimacy.

Primary respiratory muscles—having "breathing space" and fullness of being.

Secondary respiratory muscle—control of lowering and raising of energy level related to emotional change and physical exertion.

Superficial belly muscles—containing emotional and energetic digestion, feelings and visceral streaming sensations.

Psoas (either of two muscles in the abdomen and pelvis)—intimate bonding.

Quadratus lumborum—balance between acting from impulse or from one's own feelings or in response to others.

Spinal extensors—"standing tall," holding erect, ability to withstand physiological and emotional stressors.

Hip flexors—initiating forward movement and allowing sensual/intimate body contact.

Hip abductor—personal balance, sexual identity and personal boundaries (breadth of stance).

Hip rotator—social signaling, sexual/sensual self-awareness and boundaries.

Hip extensors—ability to both move powerfully forward and stop forward movement; strength to stand alone, performance durability, capacity and ability to take a fall.

Hip adductors—sexual/sensual, intimate contact and feelings.

Pelvic floor—containment of deep visceral and sexual/sensual feelings and sensations.

Tensor fascia latae, fractus iliotibialis and knee extensor—personal boundaries in close and distant relationships; collecting and controlling forward movement.

Knee flexor—choice of control, direction of forward movement.

Ankle (plantar) flexor—self-assertion, standing on one's own feet, ability to jump and take a fall.

Peronel muscle—personal balance in group interactions.

Ankle and toe extensors—willingness to receive, perceive and face reality.

Mid-foot and toe flexor—ability to sense the ground and soak up security, support and energy from that contact.

Muscle sensitive to trauma—pterogoids, splenius capitis and cervicus, sartorius, gracilis, plantaris and popliteus.

In my search for further information, I took various workshops to understand more about this energy psychology and how suitable changes in the emotional body could affect us. As is common with many workshops, the participants volunteered to be the "patients."

During one weekend workshop, a woman wanted to deal with emotions she was having around her child, whom she felt she was continually depriving of attention. No matter how much time she spent with the little girl she was plagued by the sense of needing to give more. This issue was looked at and then deprogrammed using new kinesthetic and cognitive therapies, and she was comfortable that the issue had been released. The next day, when the workshop started with a question and answer period, she asked if they could review what had happened. While she felt the emotions of the previous day had been resolved, her right forearm was now very sore, almost frozen: Was there a correlation? After identifying the muscle involved—forearm rotator, on the right side—questions were asked about her father. Yes, she had thought about her father last night; in fact, she felt that the reason she wanted to give so much attention to her child was because her father had never given her enough attention. She remembered a very distinct incident, when she was "bleeding to death" and her father failed to help her; he froze. Her emotions (of giving and receiving) were addressed by the workshop coordinator and the pain in her arm almost immediately disappeared. The forearm rotator deals with giving and receiving—closing and opening exchange, and the body's right side represents male issues, especially paternal relationships.

This dramatic example illustrated several things for me. First, that these emotions are dynamically linked, just as several psychological models have suggested. Dr. Stanislav Grof, MD (psychiatrist and Scholar-in-Residence at the Esalen Institute) explains that emotions are dynamically linked and reside outside time lines. A simple cue (like a smell, sight or circumstance) can trigger an emotion that first occurred many years earlier. Once you become aware of the simple surface emotion, often there is a more intense emotion underlying it that creates the "magnetic" pull. When the underlying emotion is revealed the release is almost instant, and when the emotion is cleared the physical symptoms are immediately healed.

Other theories go even further and suggest that these somatic symptoms are harmonics or morphic resonances of issues perceived in the more subtle bodies. The old profound statement "As above, so below" comes to mind. Again, I see that not only are emotions (astral body, above) frozen into the muscle and viscera of the body (below) to be dealt with at a later time, but these frozen muscles are in themselves just symptoms of emotional anomalies or energy patterns that cloud the emotional body. I found that while body work like Rolfing and Trager were releasing emotions, they were dealing primarily with the somatic complaints. Flower essences, homeopathic remedies, drop-level herb therapy and possibly some of the new tapping kinesiology therapies I was looking at could release the emotional issues, and thus also clear the physical symptoms.

Oral dose items: herbs, flower essences and homeopathics

As explained in the previous two chapters, there are several oral dose products that have been found beneficial for working on the transformation of emotional issues. There is nothing wrong (in fact it is quite common) in working with more than one body at a time. Herbals, elixirs, homeopathics and flower essences can all be given at the same time.

I like to think of many of the oral dose remedies as forms of positive, physical affirmation of what transpired in the treatment room. These oral dose remedies have great function in themselves, but also anchor the person back to the communication that transpired during the treatment session. This can be an effective means of focusing the astral body in the transformation process. See the Repertory section for lists of suggested oral dose products to use.

Creativity without perfectionism

For many of my patients, a daily dose of fifteen minutes filled with creativity—without perfection—can turn around some dramatic health issues: this is a simple and basic technique with profound effects.

When I created the analogy of emotional roughage, I realized the emphasis was on the need to release or eliminate unwanted emotional material, and the best release mechanism, for emotionally sensitive individuals, is creative expression. Two of the expressive tools I initially recommended were knitting and cross-stitching—rhythmic and "earth bound." Not long after starting the technique, I noticed that some were taking the whole creativity process far too seriously for therapeutic purposes and in fact, were turning the practice into a major project.

Consequently, I asked those who were not improving to bring their creative project to the next visit. Certainly they were being creative and had clearly taken my instructions to heart: there were elaborate sweater designs, complex cross-stitching patterns, and amazingly detailed paintings, almost all "masterpieces." Even though most of the projects looked fabulous, many a creator said, "it really isn't that good." Seemingly, they were afraid I would give them a low grade, even though that was not my function—this was an exercise and therapy for emotional release, not an art class.

The quest was on to fine-tune a technique that would provide for those patients who were also perfectionists. Cross-stitching was out, it was far too detailed. I tried using creative modalities that were removed from their real talents—so painters wrote and writers sketched. Those who commuted on rapid transit were asked to knit a simple scarf on the way in, and unravel it on the way back. At first, this was very frustrating for them, but it did yield results; apparently the rhythm of creating and releasing was the crucial factor, not the scarf itself.

As a herbalist/biologist, one of the questions I often ask myself is, "How does this problem relate to our distant ancestors' lifestyle?" The answer helps me determine what may be "hard-wired" into the human system. Historically, humans were creative out of necessity; for example, if they wanted to carry berries back to camp, they had to weave a basket. However, once all survival needs were met by a group, creative expression remained central to all cultures because it fulfills both physical and psychological drives.

The idea with this therapy is to engage in a process that is releasing. Many feel that taking classes will assist with their creativity. However, formal training can often increase anxiety and reduce the creative drive—especially for those who feel compelled to paint the perfect picture or play the perfect melody. Self-criticism impedes the creative flow, therefore improvisational classes such as dancing and drumming facilitate personal expression and better encourage creativity.

As mentioned earlier, other types of release, such as doodling, painting, keeping a journal, writing a poem, singing, chanting or any activity that creates a flow and requires little mental processing, is constructive. Stress, tension and worry dissolve and help us access a different part of ourselves.

Often people suggest reading as a means to turn off the mental chatter in their head. Unfortunately, as good as reading is for expanding your intellectual horizons, that is still more input. We need output here—output with no judgment attached to what is coming out. Even though some could argue that reading stimulates imagination and creates pictures in the mind's eye (which is good), we are looking for releasing emotions into environment. Writing these images in a journal would be a good form of release.

The rhythm of drums and percussion instruments seems to be very therapeutic, the only drawback being that some learning is required before an uninterrupted flow can be achieved. Drumming provides a good, nonverbal focus for adolescents with attention-deficit disorder/attention-deficit hyperactivity disorder (ADD/ADHD), moving them out of mind chatter and hyperactivity into mindfulness, a relaxed and centered state. When a person begins drumming, total concentration is required in order to learn the count of a rhythm; eventually, muscle memory takes over and repeating the rhythm takes less work. Once the muscles and mind have learned the kinesthetic of the rhythm, the drumming itself becomes a form of meditation.

Movement and dance are also therapeutic. For example, Gabrielle Roth, a dancer from New York City, offers improvisational movement workshops to people around the world. She has developed a system of free movement for five core rhythms from which individuals of all ages and from all walks of life may benefit. Roth's book, *Sweat Your Prayers: The Five Rhythms of the Soul*, extols the benefits of creative movement.

Energy psychology

We have found with cases of chronic fatigue or fibromyalgia that sometimes everything seems to be unfolding and healing nicely when suddenly a patient seems to reach an impasse and occasionally has a complete relapse. These stumbling blocks can happen with any type of therapy.

To borrow a concept from the homeopaths, these blocks are like miasms, many of which I have found to be emotional; whether unresolved trauma, fear, anxiety, phobia, loss, addiction, obsession or compulsion. Consequently, these past, unresolved traumas or intense negative emotional experiences may act as miasms or blocks on the road to recovering health. Chronic fatigue syndrome and fibromyalgia, in particular, are associated with post-traumatic stress syndrome. I have investigated some of the new therapies known as "energy psychology" to determine if they can correct these retained stress experiences.

The purpose of energy psychology is to treat psychological issues consistently, in quantum leaps, without the need to pass through often lengthy stages of discovery, emoting and cognitive restructuring that are often found in some types of psychotherapy. The idea here is not to discredit these longer forms of therapy, but, in some cases, therapy can be done more quickly, so why not? The objective of energy therapy is to identify various disruptive energy configurations that can be acknowledged and then quickly and simply dispatched. Energy psychology is also used in areas such as peak performance, education, vocational sports and industrial psychology.

While psychological issues manifest behaviorally, cognitively, neurologically and chemically, they really start as an energy pattern. Often by finding the energy pattern, we can affect the first domino in the cascade of events that causes the behavior. Because emotions are rooted in energy configurations in the emotional body, psychological phenomena are fundamentally quantum mechanic events or processes. Negative emotions exist at low levels of inertia as compared to matter. Since energy is not highly inert, psychological issues can be resolved more easily than originally thought. It is merely a matter of altering the energy field. So, instead of long counseling sessions that take sixty minutes a week for months or even years, these energy psychology sessions can make changes in one or two sixty-minute sessions.

There are several types of energy psychology therapies currently being used in North America. We suggest three that have been clinically tested and reported on in the academic literature: visual/kinesthetic dissociation (V/KD) (Bandler and Grinder, 1979); eye movement desensitization and reprocessing (EMDR) (Shapiro, 1995) and thought field therapy (TFT) (Callahan, 1983).

Follow-up of the therapies within the four- to six-month range revealed that all of these approaches yielded sustained reduction in subjective units of stress (SUD)—which are rated by the subjects themselves upon reviewing the traumatic memories. Any of the following methods effectively reduces distress associated with trauma, including nightmares, intrusive recollections and phobic responses.

Visual/Kinesthetic Dissociation (V/KD)

During this type of therapy, the client is asked to dissociate from the ill feeling associated with a trauma memory, a phobia or any negative emotion–inducing situation, by reviewing the event from an altered visual perspective.

There is more than one approach to V/KD; a common method is to get the client to visualize sitting in a theater, watching a black and white snapshot, just before the scene of trauma. With this scene in mind, the therapist asks for the next level of disassociation by saying, "And now float out of your body seated there in the theater and float back here in the projection booth with me while we watch you down there seated in the theater, watching the younger you, way over there in the past on the movie screen. And continue to remain safely and comfortably up here in the projection booth with me, as we observe you seated in the theater, watching the movie of the traumatic event unfold in slow motion."

The client is asked to let the scene unfold, until it is over and the client feels relatively safe, allowing the scene to freeze into a snapshot. Next the client is asked to re-associate into the seated position in the theater: "And now float back down into your body seated there in the theater, continuing to observe that snapshot of the safe scene after the trauma is over."

After this phase is completed, the client is asked to associate into the scene on the screen: "And now step into the safe moment up on the screen. I am going to ask you to do something that only sounds difficult as I describe it, but you will actually find it fairly easy to do. When I say "begin," allow the scene to become colorful and to rapidly proceed backward all the way to the beginning. Everything should be going in reverse: gestures, walking, moving, words and so on. Allow this all to happen very quickly, taking no more than two or three seconds to complete. And when you are at the beginning of the scene, that safe place before it all began, I would like you to stop picturing the scene and to look out at me. Do you understand? Ready? Begin."

After checking the client's emotional response, the therapist will decide if the process needs to be repeated, up to a few more times, until the distress disappears. This technique comes out of Neuro-Linguistic Programming (NLP) developed by Bandler and Grinder and has had a strong following since the late 1970s.

Eye Movement Desensitization and Reprocessing (EMDR)

EMDR directs the client to review traumatic memories while "tracking" eye movements in response to the therapist's prompts. The client is also asked to think negative beliefs (e.g., "I'm powerless") at the beginning of the process and sometimes intermittently during the eye movement process. The client is asked to pay attention to physical and emotional factors stimulated through the process. The practitioner promotes eye movement when subjective units of distress (SUD) emerge. During this process, a significant reduction of SUD will be noticed and positive beliefs (e.g., "I'm worthwhile") are introduced during eye movement to "install" beliefs. Throughout this process, greater memory networks of the trauma incident often emerge and are dealt with. The client is asked if there are problems found in other locations by including a "body scan" directive to evaluate the process. Other forms of stimulus including tones, light and physical tapping are sometimes used.

Shapiro believes that the stimulations trigger "a physiological mechanism that activates the information-processing system." She goes on to explain its mechanism of action referring to "... a differential effect of neuronal bursts caused by various stimuli, which may serve as the equivalent of a low-voltage current and directly affect synaptic potential; [and] de-conditioning caused by a relaxation response." It is thought that this is a natural process and usually happens in lesser issues, but gets blocked in more traumatic issues. The EMDR serves to activate this natural healing mechanism as might be seen in dream states.

Thought Field Therapy (TFT)

TFT directs the client to focus on disturbing traumatic memories or other emotionally charged conditions while physically tapping on specific acupuncture meridian points. The therapist starts out with a diagnostic process that involves muscle testing (applied kinesiology) to determine a specific sequence of meridian points needing activation in order to achieve therapeutic results.

The client is asked to review the traumatic memory, rating the subjective units of distress (SUD) between 1 and 10, then briefly taps on each of the potent meridian points in sequence (e.g., beginning of an eyebrow above the bridge of the nose, directly under an eye orbit, approximately 4 inches under the armpit and under the collarbone, next to the sternum). The SUD rating is taken again, which has usually dropped. Then, another tapping sequence is done—the Nine Gamut Treatment (9G): simultaneously tapping between the little finger and the ring finger on the back of the hand while moving eyes (closed then open) down left and down right, eyes in a clockwise and counterclockwise motion, humming notes, counting and humming again. The traumatic incident is reviewed again, usually with a further lowering of SUD. The whole process is repeated if the SUD is not at 1.

Often during this process, associated memories come to the surface that are dealt with in the same manner. In some clients, no result is seen at first, and this is considered a psychological reversal (PR), which is blocking the process. It is believed that the flow in the meridians is in the wrong direction. This energy pattern results in a process whereby the client unconsciously sabotages the treatment process. A PR treatment usually fixes this and then the above procedure is repeated, getting the desired results. Many types of PR treatments have evolved, but one of the most commonly used ones is simply tapping on the little finger side of the hand while repeating an affirmation such as, "I accept myself even though I have this problem."

TFT is based on the concept that psychological issues are manifestations of isolative active information energetically coded within the thought fields. Callahan defines the thought field as "… the specific thoughts, perturbations and related information which are active in a problem or threat situation. In order to diagnose and treat effectively, the appropriate thought field must be attuned." These thought fields can be a phobic object or traumatic memory. A perturbation is defined as "the fundamental and easily modifiable trigger containing specific information which sets off the physiological, neurological, hormonal chemical and cognitive event, which results in the experience of specific negative emotions." By removing the perturbation(s) from the thought field, traumatic experience is alleviated and released.

At our clinic, we have a number of practitioners on staff who have been trained in the TFT process. The results we see give us the confidence that it is the most suitable method for our health practitioners and doctors, from many disciplines, to use. This does not mean that we do not refer clients to professionals trained exclusively in psychological or counseling therapies; in fact we have a registered psychologist on staff. We find that TFT helps move some patients through the emotional blocks or miasms, so we can get back to our other modalities of healing. Clearly, there are many other types of counseling that are appropriate for other types of problems.

The first case treated with TFT was by Callahan in 1980. He had a female patient in her forties who had suffered from a life-long phobia of water for which she had already been in therapy for a year; he had tried a variety of traditional approaches with no results. With TFT, this phobia was eliminated by a treatment that took less than a minute (Callahan, 1996); and she has since had no recurrences of her phobia.

In review, TFT treatment consists of stimulation of (usually by tapping) a precise sequence of acupuncture meridian points on the body. TFT proposes and demonstrates through its successful procedures that the meridian system, when addressed with precision, provides the basis for the control system of the disturbing emotions and, more generally, for healing. When the appropriate encoded form for each disturbing emotion is addressed, rapid and complete results typically ensue.

How does this work? One possibility is that tapping on specific acupuncture points, in a certain sequence, seems to set up a frequency at both the vibrational level of the living matrix and living crystal level. Are we tapping a code into the physical body's system and using our own living matrix and living crystal system to transmit this information into the astral and mental body? It seems probable to me. This communication is not only one way; apparently, Callahan has come across the combination or set of "passwords" to the aid in that communication.

I like to think of our body as a radio receiver, and the living crystal and living matrix as the functional part of the receiver. The TFT algorithms are like dialing up specific radio stations. By going through Callahan's sequence we access a specific thought field and can discharge the negative influences they may be having in our lives.

Creative visualization

I have learned the most about the transformative power of imagery from Claudette Melchizedek, who runs an organization called the Blue School, which is based on the ancient Jewish alchemical mystery school tradition. This high-spirit woman uses the realm of images to help people get in better touch with emotions and show us how to connect to the emotional side of being. She works with images in much the way one would work with dreams. Using them as a symbolic language, we can focus on these personal images and use them to create positive emotional experiences. Claudette is married to Drunvalo Melchizedek of Flower of Life and Mer-Ka-Ba meditation fame, for people who follow that area of esoteric study. She uses many techniques of guided imagery to do emotional work. The Blue School techniques that I use the most in the clinic are reversing exercise and transforming choices.

Reversing exercise is extremely simple but quite profound. Elders of the Blue School believe that if only this exercise is practised, it can transform a person's whole emotional life. It is considered a window into the world of dreams and aids in using that world to transmute emotions on the level of the astral body. Because of this, it is best done before bed.

Every night in bed, before falling asleep, you simply go through the events of the day—in reverse; starting with the last thing done before going to bed, and ending with the first event of the day. Pay special attention to emotional incidences you see in your mind's eye as you reverse the day; save positive incidences and erase negative ones. Micro-details of the day (e.g., unbrushing your teeth) are not required; the day is scanned for personal life events. Many of my patients find that, at first, they fall asleep before they finish the process. This is quite normal. As time goes on, reversing back to the morning becomes much easier.

This process helps open up the dream world and makes it clearer. To take an analogy from the computer world, I like to think of the reversing exercise as a defragmenting program, something that cleans up your hard drive and helps it run more efficiently. The reversing process is like defragmenting your emotional body before it runs the dream time programs.

Also, this technique helps integrate communication with the emotional realm, via the chakra system, especially the fourth, or heart chakra. An add-on to the reversing exercise is, after you reverse events back to the morning, to imagine a white light shining out of the body's pores and connecting to the universe, just before falling asleep.

The reversing exercise can be done anytime during the day, to aid in reversing out problems that have come up. After you become proficient, it will assist with going beyond the day and dealing with issues that occurred much earlier in life.

Transforming choice through the right use of will—I have modified and simplified this Blue School exercise to suit my patient load. It is made up of six parts.

1. Transforming choices: Each month choose one tendency or emotion that you wish to transform. Identify the tendency or emotion by name, muscle group associated (if known, refer to the muscle chart earlier in this chapter) and if there is an associated color or sound, add it. Identify the feeling and transpose it to the opposite feeling. If the opposing feeling is unknown or unidentified, transform it into love.

Feeling of lack of self-worth	Loving self
Brownish color	Radiant blue
Pectoral and chest muscles	Expand chest muscles

I suggest patients imagine which colors are appropriate and visualize the associated muscle if known. They are asked to do this twice a day, usually in the morning after they have showered, and in the evening before going to bed. The corresponding flower essence associated with the particular emotional issue might also be given. Sometimes, herbal remedies and homeopathics, if applicable, may be taken to strengthen the visualization exercise. A more extended affirmation, as found in the Louise Hay material, may also be added.

2. Time table: Women start at the end of one menstrual cycle, stop at the first sign of the next menstruation and start the next cycle when that menstruation ends. Men start at the new moon and stop twenty-one days later, starting the cycle again at next new moon.

3. Reversing exercise is done nightly before going to bed, paying special attention to the current month's tendency or emotion.

4. Attentiveness and change during the day is achieved by staying alert for the first sign of the current month's emotional tendency to arise during the day. As an example: if a person is working with the emotion impatience, he or she would try to observe whenever impatience arises in their day-to-day life. Efforts to reverse the emotion or tendency can be made either during or immediately after its occurrence. Failure to do so is no cause for alarm and is considered quite normal. As the month progresses, the emotion is liable to arise more— a natural tendency as this emotion is cleansed from the body. The process might be called an emotional healing crisis. What cannot be achieved during a specific day can be tried again at night (see 3).

5. Stopping (as in 2). Women stop at the first stage of menstruation and men twenty-one days after the new moon

6. Next month: Regardless of whether or not the previous month's emotion has been dealt with (it can always be revisited), a new tendency or emotion should be started.

Practicing this technique for about six months will result in the ability to identify and transform an emotion when it first appears.

The sabotage

In the endeavor to erase emotional miasms and emotions trapped in muscles, it is necessary to reconnect with the healthy flow of emotions that link energy to the chakras via the etheric body. However, the self-healing process is often sabotaged by the presence of mental chatter—which is impatient and demands instant results. Remember, these emotions took a long time to evolve; they will not be solved in a day, week or month. Often the mental chatter takes over and tries to convince that there is no time for this process work. Quiet the chatter and the time will be found.

Think of the process, regardless of how many times it is started and restarted, as planting a seed: it takes time to germinate, grow and bear fruit. In order to grow, the seedling must be irrigated with the water of positive emotion. Not all seeds germinate, nor do all seedlings bear fruit, but if we keep planting the seeds, sooner or later we will reap the fruits.

Mindfulness

While there are botanicals like reishi or skullcap to help quell mind talk, the practice of mindfulness will do wonders. Mindfulness is the process that begins purification of the mind. The whole concept comes from the Buddhist traditions, and it is used by some medical doctors, like Dr. Dacher, to treat PNI-related health issues.

This healing practice works as soon as the mind becomes an observer instead of a participant—on automatic pilot engaged in mind. Mindfulness consists of consciously choosing to detach from the event or scene that is going on and engage as a witness. We still feel and experience emotions, but now we are able to be in our life with attention. For example, the mind observes the presence of anxiety in a situation and, instead of identifying and reacting with anxiety, the emotion is consciously observed: detachment diffuses the emotion. With practice and patience, mindfulness can take us beyond the conventional definition of health to what Dacher coins, "super health." The mind is still, the heart open, and we see and experience what is happening here and now. Although from time to time we might all experience this state, the goal is to maintain these moments of tranquility and well-being for longer and longer periods.

CHAPTER NINE

Beginning to Heal

So, what have we learned so far? Healing from the perspective of vibrational energy can be explained and summarized as follows:

1. Our physical body is much more integrated than originally thought by the scientific community just a few years ago. Autoimmune issues arise when any one part of the body attacks another part. The living cellular matrix connects all parts of the body from the nucleus of every cell to the structural network of the entire body. The body comprises many living crystals that work as communication devices and can receive and store electromagnetic information. Many of the body's functions work by entrainment mechanisms and by morphic resonance. Therefore, we have to be careful to what we entrain. For the physical body, the most beneficial frequency to entrain to is Earth, Gaia or nature. For the astral body, love or the heart chakra is the most balancing entrainment.

2. Stress is a major factor in how we perceive and communicate with our world. Stress can cause blockages in our energy systems, thus creating qi stagnation and triggering many forms of autoimmune disease.

3. The science of psychoneuroimmunology (PNI) shows that the physical body functions as an integrated communication system. We have to consider it as a whole, along with its connection to the subtle bodies.

4. Emotional sensitivity and emotional "roughage" are part of our daily lives. They need to be kept in balance. Too much input without sufficient expression also results in qi stagnation, which can lead to many diseases, including autoimmune issues.

5. We are far more than our physical body. We are made up of physical, etheric, astral (emotional), mental and causal bodies, each of which vibrates at an increasingly faster frequency and has its own internally regulated set of systems, similar to the physical body. All of the bodies communicate with each other. Two of the communication systems linking the physical body with the subtle bodies are the acupuncture meridian system and the chakra system.

6. We are really holographic projections of universal energy, reflecting the electromagnetic and magnoelectric nature of our being. The function of negative entropy can be summed up as the vital energy that drives our lives and is projected into our physical body by the subtle bodies. One of the mechanisms for this projection is the chakra system. If there are blockages or qi stagnation in the various bodies, we will not receive adequate vital energy from this holographic projection. We are merely part of an eternal universe that has more dimensions than we can see in the three-dimensional world.

7. In the attempt to control the flow of "our" own world, we sometimes interrupt or constrict the flow of the vital energy emerging from the subtle bodies, which results in symptom sets and disease. The endeavor is to determine the location of these constrictions or blockages and release them.

8. There are many tools from the botanical world in the form of herbs, flower essences and homeopathics that can help to

discharge these electromagnetic and magnoelectric block-ages—which helps the body to heal instead of attacking itself. The botanical kingdom is the perfect conduit for helping us entrain to earth, Gaia and nature.

9. Counseling techniques can assist in dealing with emotional blocks and especially with emotional miasms. Emotional miasms are often major blocks to healing in autoimmune issues.

These points condense to one simple concept: the direction and balance of flow. We are transformed by the direction and balance of the flow of vital energy through our being. Pressure one way can transform a person into a different "shape" of themselves.

Most of us are trying to take in too much of our three-dimensional physical world, thus interrupting the vital essence that comes from the subtle parts of our hologram. We are constantly pulling energy into our physical body from the environment, so much so that vital energy cannot come through us. Why are we doing this? The answer is complex; however, one of the reasons appears to be a desire to increase self-esteem. Was that not the pattern of perfectionism exhibited by the chronic fatigue syndrome personality? These individuals keep themselves so busy in order to achieve a certain level of status in their environment, while all along increasingly isolating themselves from that same environment. They work progressively harder and more perfectly to obtain the elusive goal of sustainable self-esteem—from the external world—which, in reality, can come only from within. This type of self-esteem involves a clear flow of vital energy from the subtle bodies, without major blockages. With continual input from the external environment, the flow of vital energy from the subtle bodies is disrupted.

Is vital energy flow like breathing? We inhale and exhale continuously; if we only inhaled we would soon die from the toxins built up from the carbon dioxide in our body. Yes, we consume energy from our environment, food, oxygen, relationships and the awe of Earth's beauty. But we also have to balance that consumption by releasing into our environments. We absorb emotional and mental energies, as well as physical energy; therefore we must also express them—which is necessary to pull vital energy into our physical body from the subtle bodies. The idea of breath and vital essence gives us a new way of looking at physical cleanses, detoxification programs and fasting cures. They not only work to cleanse the physical body but also are energetically releasing for the subtle bodies.

Conversely, if we only exhaled and tried to get all of our energy from our subtle bodies, our physical body would eventually expire and that part of the hologram would dissolve. Accordingly, it is a two-way flow as we breathe in and breathe out the vital essences of the universe, renewing our bodies and replenishing our souls.

Remember, people with autoimmune issues start off with a strong immune system, in fact, stronger than normal. Autoimmune patients often have the strongest constitution. The immune system gets a signal to start an attack—overreacts—often resulting in attacking itself. We need to incorporate that constitutional strength into healing energy. With better communication and flow of vital energies from the subtle bodies, this situation can be reversed. First, the autoimmune situation is reduced and then, in time, resolved. If there has already been substantial damage done to the physical body, this might remain. In some incidences these too can be reversed.

The goal is to move on into a more vibrant, integrated self, one that feels comfortable with self, with clear communication between the various subtle bodies and the physical body. In Part Four of this book, the Repertory, we have listed treatment protocols for many autoimmune issues to help achieve those goals.

Afterword

❖

Let's look back and see how the protocols worked for the patients mentioned earlier.

Sabina was both working in her family restaurant and as an aspiring opera singer. Even though she was a strong healthy woman, this was too much for her. She was definitely getting the creative release she needed, but it was extremely perfectionist. She desired personal achievement and competency but the striving was too much and she had burned herself out. She took the herbs that helped build her up, but one of the most important things she did was to keep a journal. By journal writing on a regular basis, she released a lot of pent-up tension. Release was her strongest cure and helped her decide on a new life direction.

Raylin was mostly helped by the reishi mushroom supplement, as many other asthmatics have been. It aided in calming him down, and giving him a chance to realize his own emotions were part of the stress that precipitated the attacks. Raylin, unbeknownst to himself or me at the time, created his own form of mindful observation to short-circuit emotional issues before they settled into his chest.

Maria's rheumatic arthritis had to do with a combination of physical diet and emotional attitude. After doing a series of detox and cleanses, she started losing weight, which in turn gave her a stronger feeling of self-esteem, thus releasing the rheuma-toid arthritis.

Christina clearly just burnt herself out by overworking in her new law practice. One of her most significant issues was the emotional sensitivity and stress in interpersonal relationships. This combined with the heavy workload tipped the health scales. She recognized enough early signs to know she should slow down, but she was so intent on becoming partner (to increase self-esteem) she ignored them—clearly, a case of trying to get every-thing she needed from her environment without taking time to breathe. The supplements built her strength up and got her going again, but she still froze up from time to time. Christina had some early unresolved childhood trauma, an emotional miasm (around self-worth). Once that was released through thought field therapy she was able to express her normal vibrant self. We also found that making up a flower essence of pomegranate, walnut and yarrow helped her immensely. The pomegranate is for conflict between career and family, especially in women; walnut helps a person to not be influenced by others when they are going through a change; and yarrow is for sensitivity to negative influ-ence and to develop stronger personal boundaries (5 drops, 3 times a day).

George's high blood pressure certainly had to do with his diet and his stress-coping skills. While the herbs relaxed him and helped regulate his blood pressure, anger and other stresses brought it right back up again. Once he learned how to deal with his anger and other frustrations, he slowly decreased the supple-ments, and is now some 35 pounds lighter.

Cindy's irritable bowel syndrome was almost completely emotionally based. She needed a good inner cleanse or detox and supplements to adjust her intestinal flora, and get her elimination system back into a natural balance. Self-esteem was a big issue for her, as well as an emotional trauma from the past. Once she released the emotional miasm, some counseling sessions with a psychologist helped her rearrange her life and develop better coping skills.

The answer to my mystery: Why do some of my healthiest patients start manifesting some of the most difficult health problems?

Many of these people with chronic fatigue and autoimmune-based disorders had strong physical bodies. They often relied solely on their physical body to pull themselves through most events and experiences in life. Often they looked for physical solutions, burying their emotional issues in their muscles and astral body, slowly congesting the flow of vital energies from those areas. Since most of them were more sensitive than average, they also had more to bury. This congestion was so slow it was not noticed as it was happening. It was the straw that broke the camel's back syndrome. Or was it more like the story of the frog?

If you try to put a frog in boiling water, he will jump right out. If you put him in cool water and slowly heat it up, the frog will cook to death. Slow, continuous, low-grade stress can often be worse than short-term dramatic stress.

Again the answer was direction and balance of the flow of vital energy. Each in his or her own personal way had constricted this flow. Each in his or her own personal way found a means to shift and transform.

PART FOUR

Repertory

Vibrational Health Programs

❀

The following, by no means exhaustive, list of certain major autoimmune health problems and their remedies is provided as a means of opening up the discussion on treating these and other health issues from the vibrational perspective. The first job of the practitioner or patient is to determine in which body, or bodies, the center of gravity of the health issue is located—you might have to seek out a practitioner versed in the concepts of vibrational medicine to help you determine this. Then review which herb is most significant. We have included only problems that fall into our broadened definition of autoimmune and PNI issues. A more complete list can be found on the Web site: www.mindbodyharmony.com.

Dosages

Please note: The following information is not intended as a substitution for consultation with your physician or health care practitioner.

If the health issue is in the physical body usually the dosage is in a crude amount of 1–2 capsules, or 20 drops of tincture, twice daily. For more information on these herb dosages, or for more information on the formulas, you can refer to the extensive book I wrote on the subject: *Dr. Willard's Encyclopedia of Herbal Use*, published by Key Porter Books, or on our Web sites: www.wrc.net. or www.wildrosecollege.com. These Web sites have more thorough information on the various herbs and formulas with suitable references.

If the issue appears to be more etheric, use 1–3 drops of the fresh tincture. Again, it is most appropriate to find the energetics of the specific herb for this. I have also listed the chakra(s) that rule each of the health issues, so specific work can be done with that.

The flower essences deal mostly with the astral or emotional body, and I have listed several for each of the emotions. A review of these remedies can be found in several flower essence books. I usually refer to *Flower Essence Repertory* (FER). This list is meant only to make your referencing easier, almost like an index. Flower essences are not disease specific, the way we have listed them here. You will still have to look at the dominating emotions and select the appropriate remedy. The homeopathics are similar to the flower essences, in that what I have listed here is more like a fast index method to look up a possible homeopathic that may be appropriate. To see if the remedy truly is the right remedy, you will still need to refer to a homeopathic *materia medica* to see which one fits the symptom picture best. In several, I have listed the time-tested homeopathic formula. You might want to start with these formulas, as they are more broad spectrum. If this does not seem efficient enough you can look more specifically into the symptom details of the other homeopathic preparations. For more information on these herb dosages or for more information on the formulas, refer to the resources section at the end of this book.

Under the "other" category, we have listed several items that are advisable to try. Some of them are standard to all ailments, such as spending time in nature to entrain the emotions to earth energy.

Allergies

Physical

Herbs: Reishi, alfalfa, ma huang, freeze-dried nettles, lobelia, Reishi Plus Formula, Lung Formula.

Nutritional supplements: Digestive enzymes, BEVC, beta-carotene, vitamin C, essential fatty acids.

Chakras: Respiratory: Fourth; Digestive: Third

Flower Essences to Consider

Power issues: California pitcher plant, fairy lantern, pink yarrow.

Guilt: Elm, golden ear drops, mullein, pine, pink yarrow.

Insecurity: Aspen, baby blue eyes, evening primrose, garlic, golden yarrow, goldenrod, pink monkeyflower, rosemary, star thistle.

Barrier issues: Fawn lily, pink monkeyflower.

Sensitivity: Aspen, beech, chaparral, lavender, mountain penny-royal, mugwort, nicotiana, pink monkeyflower, pink yarrow, purple monkeyflower, yarrow.

Homeopathic

Asthmatic: Ambra grisea, argentium nitricum, arsenicum, arsenicum iodatum, cuphea, ipecac, lobelia, pulsatilla, sambucus, spongia.

Hayfever (sinuses): Allium cepa (onion), angelica, arsenicum, betonia, capsicum, kali carb, sabadilla, sambucus, solidago, teucrium.

Digestive: Angelica, arsenicum, betonia, carum, chamomile, fennel, gentiana, ginger, ipecac, lycopodium.

Formulas: Sinusitis—Kali Bichromicum, Silicea; Breathe Aid (asthma)—Kali Carbonium, Lobelia inflata, Magnesia Phosphorica, Silicea.

Others: Walks in nature, journaling, tai chi, humidifier with essential oils (pine, spruce, lavender, eucalyptus), Sacred Elixir.

Arthritis
Physical

Herbs: Cat's claw, chaparral, devil's claw, devil's club, yucca, alfalfa, aloe vera gel or juice, curcumin (anti-inflammatory); Arthritis Formula.

Nutritional supplements: Calcium, magnesium, trace minerals, glucosamine sulfate, methylsuffonylmethane, cod or halibut liver oil and essential fatty acids.

Chakras: Third and fourth

Flower Essences to Consider

Criticism: Beech, crabapple, pine, rock water, saguaro.

Flexibility: Dogwood, oak, quaking grass, rock water, willow.

Immobility: Blackberry, cayenne, iris, larch, rock rose, scleranthus, tansy, wild oat.

Resentment: Baby blue eyes, holly, oregon grape, willow.

Homeopathic

Arthritis: Apis, bryonia (pain in joints), benzoicum acid, calcarea carbonica, calcium hypophos (hands), graphite, ledum, lithium, rhus tox, ruta.

Formula: Rheumatism, Uric Acid—Natrum Phosphoricum, Ferrum Phosphoricum, Kali Sulpuricum, Silicea.

Others: Walks in nature, journaling, Sacred Elixir, Sacred Ointment; yoga for flexibility, joint mobility and deep relaxation.

Asthma

Physical

Herbs: Ma huang, cat's claw, mullein, elderberry, lobelia extract, garlic, green tea; Lung Formula, Reishi Plus Formula.

Chakra: Fourth

Flower Essences to Consider

Overwhelm: Canyon dudleya, chamomile, corn, cosmos, dill, elm, Indian pink, oak, pink yarrow, rabbitbush.

Power issues: California pitcher plant, fairy lantern, pink yarrow.

Repression: Black-eyed Susan, centaury, dandelion, evening primrose, fuchsia, golden ear drops, larch, nicotiana, pink monkeyflower, rock water.

Stress: Aloe vera, chamomile, cherry plum, dill, elm, Indian pink, lavender, pink yarrow, star of Bethlehem, vervain.

Homeopathic

Asthmatic: Ambra grisea, argentium nitricum, arsenicum, arsenicum iodatum, cuphea, ipecac, lobelia, pulsatilla, sambucus, spongia.

Others: Walks in nature, Sacred Elixir, journaling, tai chi or yoga, singing / voice work, body work (massage, etc.).

Attention-Deficit Disorder / Attention-Deficit Hyperactivity Disorder (ADD / ADHD)

Physical

Herbs: Reishi, valerian, wild oats (*Avena*); Reishi Plus Formula, Valerian Plus Formula, Children's Elixir.

Nutritional supplements: BEVC, vitamin C, alpha lipoic acid, essential fatty acids, phosphatidyl serine, GABA.

Chakras: Third and sixth

Flower Essences to Consider

Attention: Madia, Queen Anne's lace, rabbitbrush.

Centeredness: Canyon dudleya, Indian pink, red clover, rosemary.

Concentration and focus: Clematis, cosmos, pink yarrow, Queen Anne's lace, rabbitbrush, rosemary, white chestnut.

Impatience: Calendula, cosmos, impatiens, poison oak.

Homeopathic

Concentration: Belladonna, carboneum sulphuratum, chamomile, coffea, graphite, lachesis, lecithin, lycopodium, nux vomica, phosphous, silicea.

Formula: ADHD—Belladonna, Calcarea Carbonica, Chamomile, Coffea Cruda.

Others: Walks in nature, drumming, journaling, tai chi, weight lifting/training.

Bowel and colon

Physical

Herbs: Alfalfa, cascara sagrada, Turkey Rhubarb: Herbal D-tox, Lower Bowel Tonic, psyllax.

Chakras: Second and third

Flower Essences to Consider

Catharsis: Black-eyed Susan, cayenne, chaparral, fuchsia, golden ear drops, holly, scarlet monkeyflower, willow.

Purification: Chaparral, crabapple, golden ear drops, sagebrush.

Release: Angel's trumpet, bleeding heart, chamomile, cherry plum, chestnut bud, chicory, chrysanthemum, dandelion, dogwood, filaree, honeysuckle, love-lies-bleeding, mountain pennyroyal, oak, pink monkeyflower, sagebrush, white chestnut, yerba santa.

Homeopathic

Constipation: Alumina, bryonia, collinsonia, natrum mur., nux vomica, opium, plumbum.

Diarrhea: Arsenicum, China, ipecac, podophyllum, phosphoric acid, pulsatilla.

Flatulence: Argent. nit., carbo veg, chamomilla, China, lycopodium, nux vomica.

Others: Walks in nature, Sacred Elixir, journaling, tai chi, physical exercise emphasizing sit-ups, leg lifts (strengthening body core), body work.

Chronic fatigue syndrome

Physical

Herbs: Reishi, echinacea, astragalus, licorice, chlorella, essential fatty acids, St. John's wort; Reishi Plus Formula, Ener-Jazzer, Echinacea Plus Formula.

Nutritional supplements: BEVC, beta-carotene, B complex, vitamin C, zinc, malic acid, NADH, coenzyme Q_{10}.

Chakras: Third and fourth

Flower Essences to Consider

Balance: Fawn lily, goldenrod, morning glory, nasturtium, nicotiana, pomegranate, scleranthus, sunflower, vervain.

Exhaustion and fatigue: Aloe vera, California wild rose, echinacea, elm, Indian paintbrush, lavender, morning glory, nasturtium, oak, olive, peppermint, seal-heal, vervain, white chestnut, yerba santa.

Also see Devitalization, Habit Patterns, Immune disturbances, Perfectionism, Sensitivity, Vitality from Chapter 7.

Homeopathic

Fatigue: Arnica, arsenium, carbo veg, China, hux vomica, phosphoric acid.

Others: Walks in nature, Sacred Elixir, journaling, creative work, tai chi, yoga, regular mild physical exercise.

Colitis

Physical

Herbs: Alfalfa, aloe vera, boswellia, chamomile, echinacea, goldenseal root, licorice, nettles; Psyllax, Lower Bowel Tonic, Cleansing Formula, Huang Lian Su.

Nutritional supplements: Vitamin A, B complex, calcium/ magnesium, vitamin C, essential fatty acids.

Chakras: Second and third

Flower Essences to Consider

Catharsis: Black-eyed Susan, cayenne, chaparral, fuchsia, golden ear drops, holly, scarlet monkeyflower, willow.

Purification: Chaparral, crabapple, golden ear drops, sagebrush.

Release: Angel's trumpet, bleeding heart, chamomile, cherry plum, chestnut bud, chicory, chrysanthemum, dandelion, dogwood, filaree, honeysuckle, love-lies-bleeding, mountain pennyroyal, oak, pink monkeyflower, sagebrush, white chestnut, yerba santa.

Homeopathic

Constipation: Alumina, bryonia, collinsonia, natrum mur., nux vomica, opium, plumbum.

Diarrhea: Arsenicum, China, ipecac, podophyllum, phosphoric acid, pulsatilla.

Flatulence: Argent. nit., carbo veg, chamomilla, China, lycopodium, nux vomica.

Others: Walks in nature, journaling, creativity, tai chi, yoga, physical exercise including core body work such as sit-ups, crunches, leg lifts, etc.

Crohn's disease, see Colitis

Depression

Physical

Herbs: Reishi, St. John's wort, ginkgo, essential fatty acids; Reishi Plus Formula, St. John's Wort Extract Plus Formula, Ginkgo Plus Formula.

Nutritional supplements: BEVC, folic acid, phosphatidylcholine, L-5HTP, SAMe.

Chakras: Third, sixth

Flower Essences to Consider

Depression and Despair: Baby blue eyes, borage, California wild rose, chrysanthemum, elm, gentian, gorse, hornbeam, love-lies-bleeding, milkweed, mustard, olive, pine, sagebrush, Scotch broom, wild oats, wild rose, yerba santa.

Homeopathic

Depression: Aurum, argen. nit., lycopodium, medusa, natrum mur., pulsatilla.

Others: Walks in nature, counseling, journaling, creative activities, yoga, tai chi, vigorous physical exercise such as running, aerobics, massage or other body work.

Diabetes

Physical

Herbs: Fenugreek, devil's club root, cedar berries, garlic, bitter melon, gymnema, ginkgo, green tea; Glucose Formula, Syn X.

Nutritional supplements: B complex, vitamin C, vitamin E, chromium, vanadium, alpha lipoic acid, essential fatty acids, nucleic acid.

Chakra: Third

Flower Essences to Consider

Abandonment: Baby blue eyes, evening primrose, holly, mariposa lily, Oregon grape, sweet pea.

Addiction: Angelica, baby blue eyes, chamomile, chaparral, chestnut bud, morning glory, olive, peppermint, pink monkeyflower, rosemary, sagebrush, scarlet monkeyflower, self-heal, star of Bethlehem, star tulip, sunflower.

Grief: Bleeding heart, dandelion, evening primrose, fuchsia, golden ear drops, honeysuckle, sagebrush, wild rose, yerba santa.

Nostalgia: Chrysanthemum, fairy lantern, honeysuckle.

Homeopathic

Diabetes—Chimaphila umbellata, helonias, syzygium jambolanum.

Others: Walks in nature, Sacred Elixir, journaling, creativity, yoga, tai chi, physical exercise.

Fibromyalgia

Physical

Herbs: Reishi, chlorella, St. John's wort, astragalus, ginkgo, kava kava, ginger root tea, skullcap; Reishi Plus Formula, St. John's Wort Extract Plus Formula, Muscle Relaxant Formula.

Nutritional supplements: BEVC, magnesium, malic acid, coenzyme Q_{10}, dimethylglycine, MSM, essential fatty acids.

Chakras: Third and fourth

Flower Essences to Consider

Criticism: Beech, crabapple, pine, rock water, saguaro.

Flexibility: Dogwood, oak, quaking grass, rock water, willow.

Immobility: Blackberry, cayenne, iris, larch, rock rose, scleranthus, tansy, wild oat.

Resentment: Baby blue eyes, holly, Oregon grape, willow.

Balance: Fawn lily, goldenrod, morning glory, nasturtium, nicotiana, pomegranate, scleranthus, sunflower, vervain.

Exhaustion and fatigue: Aloe vera, California wild rose, echinacea, elm, Indian paintbrush, lavender, morning glory, nasturtium, oak, olive, peppermint, seal-heal, vervain, white chestnut, yerba santa.

See also Devitalization, Habit Patterns, Immune disturbances, Perfectionism, Sensitivity, Vitality from Chapter 7.

Homeopathic

Fibromyalgia: Aconite, apis, arnica, bryonia, gelsemium, rhus tox.

Others: Walks in nature, Sacred Elixir, Sacred Ointment, **Gardner** Magic cream, journaling, creativity, yoga, tai chi, mild stretching physical exercise or creative movement work.

High Blood Pressure

Physical

Herbs: Reishi, cayenne, garlic, ginger, hawthorn, elderberry; Reishi Plus Formula, Cayenne Plus Formula.

Nutritional supplements: Calcium, magnesium, multivitamins and minerals, essential fatty acids.

Chakras: Third and fourth

Flower Essences to Consider

Anxiety: Aspen, chamomile, garlic, golden yarrow, mimulus.

Competitiveness: Holly, impatiens, mountain pride, oak, penstemon, tiger lily, trillium.

Relaxation: Canyon dudleya, chamomile, dill, lavender, red chestnut, vervain, white chestnut.

Release: Chamomile, chestnut, dandelion, dogwood, evening primrose, filaree, fuchsia, honeysuckle, mountain pennyroyal, oak, sagebrush, white chestnut, yerba santa.

Stress: Aloe vera, chamomile, dill, elm, impatiens.

Homeopathic

High blood pressure: Crataegus, glomoine, natrum mur., sulfur.

Formula: High blood pressure—Catus Grandiflorus, Baryta Carbonica, Gelsemium, Glonoinum.

Others: Walks in nature, Sacred Elixir, journaling, creativity, yoga, tai chi, mild physical exercise and deep relaxation exercises.

Hypoglycemia

Physical

Herbs: Devil's club, cedar berries (pancreas); licorice root, uva ursi leaves or Siberian ginseng (adrenals), garlic; Glucose Formula, Syn X, Four Ginsengs, Devil's Club—Huckleberry.

Nutritional supplements: B complex, vitamin C, vitamin E, multivitamins and minerals, nucleic acid, zinc, chromium (picolinate).

Chakra: Third

Flower Essences to Consider

Overwhelmed: Canyon dudleya, chamomile, corn, dill, elm, hornbeam, Indian pink, lavender, pink yarrow, rabbitbrush.

Addiction: Angelica, baby blue eyes, chamomile, chaparral, chestnut bud, morning glory, olive, peppermint, pink monkey-flower, rosemary, sagebrush, scarlet monkeyflower, self-heal, star of Bethlehem, star tulip, sunflower.

Homeopathic

Diabetes—Chimaphila umbellata, helonias, syzygium jambolanum.

Others: Walks in nature, Sacred Elixir, journaling, creativity, yoga, tai chi, mild physical exercise.

Insomnia

Physical

Herbs: Reishi, hops, valerian root, passionflower, chamomile, skullcap; Valerian Plus Formula, Reishi Plus Formula, Nerve Formula, Sleeping Formula, Children's Calming Elixir.

Nutritional supplements: Folic acid (restless leg syndrome), multivitamins and minerals, multiminerals, trace minerals, calcium, magnesium, melatonin, L-5HTP.

Chakras: Third and sixth

Flower Essences to Consider

Insomnia: Aspen, black-eyed Susan, chamomile, chaparral, dill, lavender, mugwort, red chestnut, Saint John's wort, white chestnut.

Homeopathic

Insomnia: Chamomilla, cocculus, coffea, lycopodium, nux vomica, passiflora, pulsatilla.

Formulas: Insomnia—Belladonna, Coffea Cruda, Chamomilla, Hyoscyamus.

Others: Walks in nature, Sacred Elixir, journaling, creativity, yoga, tai chi, vigorous physical exercise.

Irritable Bowel Syndrome

Physical

Herbs: Alfalfa, cascara sagrada, Turkey rhubarb, chamomile, ginger root, peppermint oil (enteric-coated); burdock root, dandelion; Lower Bowel Tonic, psyllax, chlorella, fenugreek and goldenseal.

Nutritional supplements: Vitamin A, B complex, calcium/magnesium, vitamin C, essential fatty acids, pro-biotics.

Chakras: Second and third

Flower Essences to Consider

Catharsis: Black-eyed Susan, cayenne, chaparral, fuchsia, golden ear drops, holly, scarlet monkeyflower, willow.

Purification: Chaparral, crabapple, golden ear drops, sagebrush.

Release: Angel's trumpet, bleeding heart, chamomile, cherry plum, chestnut bud, chicory, chrysanthemum, dandelion, dogwood, filaree, honeysuckle, love-lies-bleeding, mountain pennyroyal, oak, pink monkeyflower, sagebrush, white chestnut, yerba santa.

Homeopathic

Constipation: Alumina, bryonia, collinsonia, natrum mur., nux vomica, opium, plumbum.

Diarrhea: Arsenicum, China, ipecac, podophyllum, phosphoric acid, pulsatilla.

Flatulence: Argent. nit., carbo veg, chamomilla, China, lycopodium, nux vomica.

Others: Walks in nature, Sacred Elixir, journaling, creativity, tai chi, yoga, vigorous physical exercise emphasizing body core strength, weight training.

Lupus

Physical

Herbs: Reishi, pau d'arco, cat's claw, garlic, goldenseal, red clover, licorice root, milk thistle, yucca; Arthritis Formula, Reishi Plus, Cleansing Formula.

Nutritional supplements: BEVC, vitamin C, zinc, multiminerals, DHEA, essential fatty acids, calcium/magnesium, L-cysteine, L-methionine, L-lysine, glucosamine sulfate, MSM.

Chakras: Second, third and fourth

Flower Essences to Consider

Anger: Black-eyed Susan, chamomile, fuchsia, impatiens, poison oak, snapdragon.

Anxiety: Aspen, chamomile, garlic, golden yarrow, mimulus.

Depression and despair: Baby blue eyes, borage, California wild rose, chrysanthemum, elm, gentian, gorse, hornbeam, love-lies-bleeding, milkweed, mustard, olive, pine, sagebrush, Scotch broom, wild oat's, wild rose, yerba santa.

Grief: Bleeding heart, dandelion, evening primrose, fuchsia, golden ear drops, honeysuckle, sagebrush, wild rose, yerba santa.

Self-esteem: Black-eyed Susan, buttercup, centaury, evening primrose, goldenrod.

Homeopathic

Lupus: Hydrocotyle, iodum, kali bichromicum, phosphorus, sepia, thyroidinum.

Others: Walks/sitting in nature, Sacred Elixir, journaling, creativity.

Manic depression/bipolar mood disorder

Physical

Herbs: Reishi, St. John's wort, ginkgo, kava, essential fatty acids; Reishi Plus Formula, St. John's Wort Plus Formula, Ginkgo Plus Formula, Nerve Formula, Valerian Night, Phosphatidylserine with Gingko Biloba.

Nutritional supplements: BEVC, B complex, vitamin C, phosphatidylcholine, L-5HTP, SAMe, NADH.

Chakras: Third and sixth

Flower Essences to Consider

Anxiety: Aspen, chamomile, garlic, golden yarrow, mimulus.

Depression and despair: Baby blue eyes, borage, California wild rose, chrysanthemum, elm, gentian, gorse, hornbeam, love-lies-bleeding, milkweed, mustard, olive, pine, sagebrush, Scotch broom, wild oats, wild rose, yerba santa.

Homeopathic

Anxiety: Aconitum, argentium nitricum, bryonia, chamomile, kali carbonicum, lycopodium, natrum muriatcum, nux vomica, sepia, veratrum viride.

Depression: Aurum, argen. nit., lycopodium, medusa, natrum mur., pulsatilla.

Others: Walks in nature, Sacred Elixir, journaling, creativity, yoga, tai chi, aerobic physical exercise such as swimming, running, sports, hiking, body work.

Pelvic inflammatory disease

Physical

Herbs—Acute stage: Goldenseal, gold thread (*Coptis*), barberry, echinacea, garlic, chlorella. After: Dong quai, black cohosh, licorice, echinacea; chlorophyll douches, Female Formula, Echinacea Plus Formula, Fenugreek and Goldenseal, Elder Berry—Larix.

Nutritional supplements: BEVC, beta-carotene, B complex, vitamin C, vitamin E.

Chakras: Second, sometimes third

Flower Essences to Consider

Sexuality: Calla lily, crabapple, dogwood, evening primrose, fairy lantern, lady's slipper, larch, manzanita, pink monkeyflower, snapdragon, sticky monkeyflower.

Homeopathic

Pelvic inflammatory disorder: Arsenicum album, kreosotium, mercurius, rhus tox.

Formula: Anti-inflammatory—Apis mellifica, bryonia, cholchicum, causticum.

Others: Walks in nature, Sacred Elixir, journaling, creativity, tai chi, yoga, physical exercise.

Syndrome X

Physical

Herbs: Fenugreek, bitter melon, reishi, garlic, gymnema, milk thistle; Syn X, Reishi plus, Digest, Devil's Club—Huckleberry.

Nutritional supplements: BEVC, vitamin C, vitamin E, CLA, essential fatty acids, alpha lipoic acid, chromium, zinc.

Chakras: Third and fourth

Flower Essences to Consider

Abandonment: Baby blue eyes, evening primrose, holly, mariposa lily, Oregon grape, sweet pea.

Addiction: Angelica, baby blue eyes, chamomile, chaparral, chestnut bud, morning glory, olive, peppermint, pink monkeyflower, rosemary, sagebrush, scarlet monkeyflower, self-heal, star of Bethlehem, star tulip, sunflower.

Grief: Bleeding heart, dandelion, evening primrose, fuchsia, golden ear drops, honeysuckle, sagebrush, wild rose, yerba santa.

Nostalgia: Chrysanthemum, fairy lantern, honeysuckle.

Overwhelmed: Canyon dudleya, chamomile, corn, dill, elm, hornbeam, Indian pink, lavender, pink yarrow, rabbitbrush.

Homeopathic

Diabetes—Chimaphila umbellata, helonias, syzygium jambolanum.

Others: Walks in nature, Sacred Elixir, journaling, creativity, yoga, tai chi, moderate to strong physical exercise.

Index